Unleashing the
healing power
of
ANIMALS

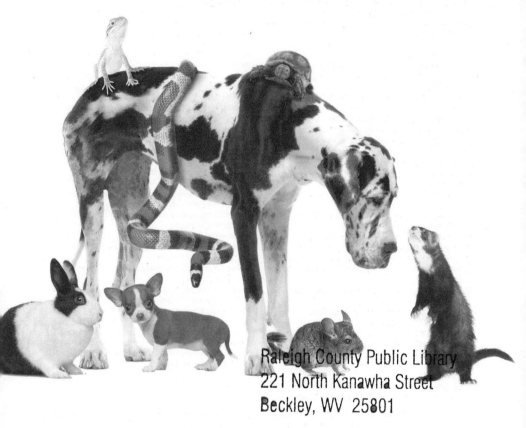

True stories about therapy animals – and what they do for us

Dale Preece-Kelly

Hubble & Hattie

The Hubble & Hattie imprint was launched in 2009 and is named in memory of two very special Westie sisters owned by Veloce's proprietors. Since the first book, many more have been added to the list, all with the same underlying objective: to be of real benefit to the species they cover, at the same time promoting compassion, understanding and respect between all animals (including human ones!) All Hubble & Hattie publications offer ethical, high quality content and presentation, plus great value for money.

More great books from Hubble & Hattie –

A puppy called Wolfie (Gregory)
Among the Wolves: Memoirs of a wolf handler (Shelbourne)
Animal Grief: How animals mourn (Alderton)
Babies, kids and dogs – creating a safe and harmonious relationship (Fallon & Davenport)
Because this is our home ... the story of a cat's progress (Bowes)
Boating with Buster – the life and times of a barge Beagle (Alderton)
Bonds – Capturing the special relationship that dogs share with their people (Cukuraite & Pais)
Camper vans, ex-pats & Spanish Hounds: from road trip to rescue – the strays of Spain (Coates & Morris)
Canne aggression – how kindness and compassion saved Calgacus (McLennan)
Cat Speak: recognising & understanding behaviour (Rauth-Widmann)
Charlie – The dog who came in from the wild (Tenzin-Dolma)
Clever dog! Life lessons from the world's most successful animal (O'Meara)
Complete Dog Massage Manual, The – Gentle Dog Care (Robertson)
Detector Dog – A Talking Dogs Scentwork Manual (Mackinnon)
Dieting with my dog: one busy life, two full figures ... and unconditional love (Frezon)
Dinner with Rover: delicious, nutritious meals for you and your dog to share (Paton-Ayre)
Dog Cookies: healthy, allergen-free treat recipes for your dog (Schöps)
Dog-friendly Gardening: creating a safe haven for you and your dog (Bush)
Dog Games – stimulating play to entertain your dog and you (Blenski)
Dog Relax – relaxed dogs, relaxed owners (Pilguj)
Dog Speak: recognising & understanding behaviour (Blenski)
Dogs on Wheels: travelling with your canine companion (Mort)
Emergency First Aid for dogs: at home and away Revised Edition (Bucksch)
Exercising your puppy: a gentle & natural approach – Gentle Dog Care (Robertson & Pope)
For the love of Scout: promises to a small dog (Ison)
Fun and Games for Cats (Seidl)
Gods, ghosts, and black dogs – the fascinating folklore and mythology of dogs (Coren)
Harry & his Grownups – A guide to training Parents (Dicks)
Helping minds meet – skills for a better life with your dog (Zulch & Mills)
Home alone – and happy! Essential life skills for preventing separation anxiety in dogs and puppies (Mallatratt)

Know Your Dog – The guide to a beautiful relationship (Birmelin)
Life skills for puppies – laying the foundation for a loving, lasting relationship (Zuch & Mills)
Lily - The dog in a million (Hamilton)
Living with an Older Dog – Gentle Dog Care (Alderton & Hall)
Miaow! Cats really are nicer than people! (Moore)
Mike&Scrabble – A guide to training your new Human (Dicks & Scrabble)
Mike&Scrabble Too – Further tips on training your Human (Dicks & Scrabble)
My cat has arthritis – but lives life to the full! (Carrick)
My dog has arthritis – but lives life to the full! (Carrick)
My dog has cruciate ligament injury – but lives life to the full! (Haüsler & Friedrich)
My dog has epilepsy – but lives life to the full! (Carrick)
My dog has hip dysplasia – but lives life to the full (Haüsler & Friedrich)
My dog is blind – but lives life to the full! (Horsky)
My dog is deaf – but lives life to the full! (Willms)
My Dog, my Friend: heart-warming tales of canine companionship from celebrities and other extraordinary people (Gordon)
Ollie and Nina and ... Daft doggy doings! (Sullivan)
No walks? No worries! Maintaining wellbeing in dogs on restricted exercise (Ryan & Zulch)
Partners – Everyday working dogs being heroes every day (Walton)
Smellorama – nose games for dogs (Theby)
The supposedly enlightened person's guide to raising a dog (Young & Tenzin-Dolma)
Swim to recovery: canine hydrotherapy healing – Gentle Dog Care (Wong)
A tale of two horses – a passion for free will teaching (Gregory)
Tara – the terrier who sailed around the world (Forrester)
The Truth about Wolves and Dogs: dispelling the myths of dog training (Shelbourne)
Unleashing the healing power of animals: True stories abut therapy animals – and what they do for us (Preece-Kelly)
Waggy Tails & Wheelchairs (Epp)
Walking the dog: motorway walks for drivers & dogs revised edition (Rees)
When man meets dog – what a difference a dog makes (Blazina)
Winston ... the dog who changed my life (Klute)
The quite very actual adventures of Worzel Wooface (Pickles)
Worzel Wooface: The quite very actual Terribibble Twos (Pickles)
Three quite very actual cheers for Worzel Wooface! (Pickles)
You and Your Border Terrier – The Essential Guide (Alderton)
You and Your Cockapoo – The Essential Guide (Alderton)
Your dog and you – understanding the canine psyche (Garratt)

Also by Dale Preece-Kelly: *Organic Guinea Pig's Health Revolution*   Photo page 35 courtesy Amanda Ravenall, *Perfect Poses Photography*

www.hubbleandhattie.com

First published May 2017 by Veloce Publishing Limited, Veloce House, Parkway Farm Business Park, Middle Farm Way, Poundbury, Dorchester, Dorset, DT1 3AR, England. Fax 01305 250479/email info@hubbleandhattie.com/web www.hubbleandhattie.com. ISBN: 978-1-845849-56-6 UPC: 6-36847-04956-0 ©Dale Preece-Kelly & Veloce Publishing Ltd 2017. All rights reserved. With the exception of quoting brief passages for the purpose of review, no part of this publication may be recorded, reproduced or transmitted by any means, including photocopying, without the written permission of Veloce Publishing Ltd. Throughout this book logos, model names and designations, etc, have been used for the purposes of identification, illustration and decoration. Such names are the property of the trademark holder as this is not an official publication.
Readers with ideas for books about animals, or animal-related topics, are invited to write to the editorial director of Veloce Publishing at the above address. British Library Cataloguing in Publication Data – A catalogue record for this book is available from the British Library. Typesetting, design and page make-up all by Veloce Publishing Ltd on Apple Mac. Printed in India by Replika Press.

Contents

Dedication 4

Preface 4

Foreword 6
by Dr Daniel Allen

1 The author 7

2 Beanz – The Border Collie 13

3 Sebastian – The Chinchilla 21

4 Mooch – The Monitor Lizard 28

5 Wasabi – The African Pygmy Hedgehog 35

6 Frostie – The Corn Snake 40

Picture Gallery 45

7 George – The Hermann's Tortoise 53

8 Tinkerbell – The Rabbit 58

9 Shiver – The Blue-Tongued Skink 63

10 Johnnie – The Ferret 67

11 And then there are 'The Others' 73

Epilogue 80

Testimonials 86

Index 88

Dedication

Lulu – 'the girl next door,' who passed away, sadly, after this book was written.

And to anyone who has ever rescued an animal, as well as all of the animals both rescued and in need of rescue worldwide. It's amazing the difference that one person can make to an animal.

Even more amazing is the difference that one animal can make to a person.

Preface

The author and publisher wish to make the reader aware of the following –

We take the subject matter of this book very seriously, and appreciate that the suitability of some of the animals for therapy work may be questioned. I understand that some of the animals I employ in my therapy work are not conventional therapy or assistance animals: I was the first to embark on working with this variety of species in a true therapy environment, which is why I am considered a pioneer in the field of animal assisted therapy. The suitability or otherwise of any species for this kind of work is subjective, although I feel that every animal has a role to play in this area.

For example, I have found in my exploration of animal assisted therapy that each animal has a different potential therapeutic effect on each person. I have also found that each person's choice of therapy animal is as unique as they are: those with no affinity to dogs, for instance, may take to a skunk or a chinchilla. I have discovered that some animals can quieten the voices in the head of a schizophrenic, and reptiles who calm and relax a psychotic ... and that's not to mention what they can do for self-esteem. Even insects can play a part in helping those with ASD (autism spectrum disorder) and hypersensitive skin.

None of my animals ever suffers as a result of the work they do – I love them too much to allow this to happen. All of the animals who work with me in therapy – regardless of species – have proven therapeutic value, and are suited to the work they do.

In researching animals who may be of benefit in my field of work I have determined that some are *not* suitable. Despite pressure to work with such animals – from patients and mental health professionals – I have always refused to do so, explaining why they would be unsuitable.

Indeed, some of the animals who live with me do not have the right temperament for my work, so therefore never attend sessions, but remain with me as companions. Vets who have assessed my animals tell me they are amongst the healthiest and most well adjusted they have seen.

All of the animals in my care have free choice about what they do, and their safety and welfare is paramount. If an animal decides to call time on the session, then that's what happens, without exception. The patients and mental health professionals I work with all realise, accept, and respect this.

Before they go into a therapy environment, I spend a long time working with my animals in order to assess their suitability for the work (some I am still working with after three years, if for no other reason than to encourage a healthy relationship with me). My animals are not 'trained,' nor made to do anything they do not want to. They are shown only love and respect, and I have a close and strong bond with each and every one of them. They are my family. During this initial process, and henceforth, they become desensitised to different environments and to being handled, which allows for a relaxed animal.

All of the animals enjoy being handled, and I am present at all times to ensure this is correctly done. This truly is as much therapy for them as it is for the patient, because all, at some point in their lives, have been mistreated, but are now in a loving, happy relationship with me, trusting me 100% to keep them safe and provide for their welfare.

I am constantly on hand during sessions, and totally aware of the animal's body language and what it tells me, which allows me to determine whether the animal is happy and relaxed, or tense and unhappy, and in danger of becoming stressed. If my animals suffered in any way, shape or form because of my work I would immediately stop doing it, and find another career! Of course, if they weren't doing the therapy work, it's possible they would simply remain caged all day, every day, which, to me, causes suffering. Because of the work we do they are not caged, and have freedom in different environments, allowing them to display natural behaviours, whilst interacting with other animals – human and non-human – at the same time.

An animal who is stressed or otherwise suffering could well use their instinctive fight or flight reflex to bite, maybe, or attempt to escape a situation, but since I began working in this way in 2010, I have never had an instance where an animal has resorted to aggression, or any behaviour indicative of suffering.

I hope that you enjoy my book, and get from it a sense of how my animals not only help the people they work with, but just how much they themselves benefit from what they do.

Dale Preece-Kelly

Foreword

Memories make us who we are. They make us individuals. Past experiences and encounters with particular animals inform our attitudes towards them, and influence emotional connections. Our relationship with any given species is interwoven with particular times in our lives.

Dale Preece-Kelly first caught my attention on social media in 2011. His zest for life and endearing updates about his ever-increasing menagerie always made me smile. When we met, I was surprised to discover that, only a year before, Dale had suffered a heart attack, lost his job, had low self-esteem, and no idea how to support his family. Remarkably, animals helped turn around Dale's life.

On the chance suggestion of a primary school teacher, Dale took his enthusiasm for animals to the next level by turning it into a successful business. Initially providing services to schools and the general public for education, he went on to work with mental health patients, delivering an innovative brand of animal assisted therapy with occupational therapists and psychologists.

Animal assisted therapy (AAT) is known to help uncover unique associations, trigger positive memories, and momentarily make us change the way we think and feel. Recognizing that individuals have complex relationships with animals, Dale saw beyond the therapeutic benefits of traditional animal companions, 'unleashing the healing power' of chinchillas, lizards, African pygmy hedgehogs, snakes, tortoises, rabbits, ferrets, skunks, and other exotic creatures.

Unleashing the healing power of animals is a personal journey: a blend of memories, experiences and encounters. It demonstrates the power of the human-animal bond; how specific relationships with individual animals can change lives, and a passion and commitment to helping others as a facilitator of animal assisted therapy. The book is a warm-hearted and uplifting read, and useful insight into the challenges and rewards of being an animal assisted therapy practitioner.

Dr Daniel Allen
Animal Geographer, and founder of Pet Nation

1
The author

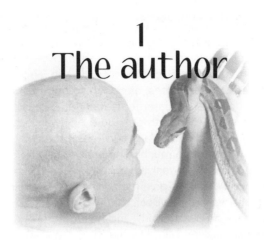

I was born in Staffordshire on April 3, 1968, and by the age of ten had developed a real love for animals, despite being bitten by the family dog. I recovered, although, sadly, our dog was 'sent to the farm' (the euphemism for euthanasia used at that time). Almost unbelievably, it wasn't until I reached my forties, with children around me, that I realised what it really meant: all those years, I'd imagined that Rusty was running around on a farm, happily helping the farmer with his daily tasks!

The animal I became particularly fond of during those early years was the rabbit. The well-known film about rabbits, *Watership Down*, was released then, and featured a rather good soundtrack by Art Garfunkel (of Simon and Garfunkel fame) and Mike Batt, the title being *Bright Eyes*. I actually received the album for Christmas that year (but if you are younger than 25 you probably won't remember records).

My love affair with rabbits was long and enduring: I loved rabbits – any kind of rabbits – and read all of the books, and spoke to breeders and keepers in order to learn everything I possibly could about them. I did my research the hard way, in a library, poring over books and making handwritten notes: how things have changed in recent years with the internet and search engines!

On my eleventh birthday I was taken in the car to collect my present, which was, you guessed it, a rabbit that my mum had reserved for me in our local pet store. Talk about 'Bright Eyes' – I was so happy with my black-and-white Dutch rabbit, who I named Silky on account of his very soft, smooth fur. I still remember the conversation I had with the store owner. I was very excited and he was very encouraging, once he had determined my knowledge of rabbits, of course. Coincidentally, around 30 years later I was selling packaging as a job, and his shop was on my round. Calling in I was delighted to find the same guy serving at the counter: he didn't remember me, but I told him all about Silky, anyway!

I joined the British Rabbit Council, and became a member of my

Unleashing the healing power of animals

local group, which held regular shows, and I began to take Silky to these, as well as others. My parents were pretty cool about it; my dad made me a carry-box to transport Silky, and they took me all over the Midlands to show my pet in competitions. He did pretty well, too, and claimed many 1st, 2nd and 3rd prizes and rosettes, although sometimes there were only two or three rabbits in class! Apparently, it was not a foregone conclusion, in these instances, that any of the three would be awarded a prize, so Silky had to be of a certain quality. I was a proud rabbit daddy.

Why did I love rabbits so much? The answer is simple: their mouth gives the impression that they wear a happy smile, and I love happy animals! And Silky would always give me a little kiss on my nose, which felt lovely. I soon discovered, however, that if I approached his hutch too quickly or loudly, this would scare him, and he would quickly turn and eject or flick urine (as male rabbits do when they are scared), and I would get a faceful of it! Learning from this my approach became slow, steady and quiet, and I always made sure that I filled his food bowl before I went in for the kiss (a ploy that later served me well with girlfriends, except that I exchanged the food bowl for a wine glass!).

I had several rabbits, but Silky was always the one I had a special relationship with. He was my pal and I shared everything with him: my hopes and dreams; my failures and hurts. At the start of my day, after breakfast, I went to feed and talk to my rabbit. At the end of my day, I would dump my bag in my room, and run to Silky to talk to him about my day. I confided in him, he knew my every secret – the girls I fancied at school; what I thought of my teachers. He knew about those who bullied me, and helped me through my tears and self-esteem issues. That rabbit was my best friend and so important to me. I used to sing him a song from the Art Garfunkel album. It's called *Oh How Happy*, and it *is* a happy tune.

I was 21 when Silky passed away, and it was one of the saddest days of my life. I had moved away from home by this time, and he had become ill with myxomatosis: a horrible, man-made disease prevalent in our wild rabbit population. There wasn't a vaccine for it back then; nor was there any treatment. My vet tried his hardest over the course of a few days to help Silky fight the disease, but to no avail.

The day Silky was to be put to sleep, I sat with him for ages before we went to the vet. I told him what was happening and explained why. I shared memories with him of all of the wonderful times we had enjoyed together, and told him how much I loved him, explaining to him that he would always be in my thoughts. It was a harrowing experience, because when I gently placed him in his box for the last time, Silky knew, and let out an ear-piercing squeal. This memory has stayed with me, and still makes me cry.

I cried for days afterwards; every thought of him brought tears. He had been everything to me.

Looking back, Silky was, albeit unknowingly, my first experience of a therapy animal. He got me through my hardest times at school – the comprehensive (High School) years. My worries about tests and exams, the highs and lows of my 'love life,' the bullies, etc. I would sit with him and pet him whilst I talked to him, which soothed my angst, made all of the bad stuff go away, and allowed me to be happy again. At the time, of course, I didn't appreciate how Silky was helping me: now, I not only fully understand how this amazing connection works, I make a living from it.

I firmly believe that the most important gift we can give a child is unconditional love, which they can receive and fully embrace, hopefully without pressure. Unfortunately, as people, our words and actions sometimes apply pressure, which an animal never does. Animals teach children how to love and how to show affection (and receive it); they teach social skills and bestow social confidence (at eleven, I felt more socially confident in the presence of other children at rabbit shows than I did in the presence of my peers at school, because we had that commonality). Animals teach us about responsibility and caring, and even, in some ways, personal hygiene (insofar as they need regular cleaning and grooming); they also teach lessons about life – when an animal is neutered, for instance, we can explain the reasons for this, and maybe even have 'the talk.'

The final – and, perhaps, most important – lesson they teach, of course, is the lesson that life, as we know it, comes to an end at some point, and how we should try and deal with it.

Many of these benefits also apply in the field of animal assisted therapy.

When it comes to acquiring a companion animal, timing is obviously relevant. It's senseless to give a three-year-old a boa constrictor, for example, as the animal needs to be age-appropriate, and suitable for a child to bond with.

My parents never became involved with Silky's care – he was *my* pet and *my* responsibility. This is an important lesson for a child to learn, and, if not, then the responsibility for the animal rests with you.

In the years following Silky's demise, my interest in animals became a little more exotic in nature, and I began to keep animals who were a little different. At this time, (the 1980s) these animals could not be found in the usual places, and the retail outlets were more often backstreet than high street.

Fast forward 20 years to 2010 and my first experience with poor health: a heart attack. It wasn't nice, I can tell you. My animal family consisted of a cat or two, a dog, a hamster, a rabbit, two guinea pigs, a bearded dragon, and a snake. Married with three stepchildren, these were our family pets. As usual, I turned to the animals around me for comfort, and the peace they have always brought me.

A few months later, I was with my youngest stepchild at his nursery interview. He was enthusing to the teacher about all of our animals, telling her all about them. She listened intently to him. At the end of the interview, she took me to one side and suggested that I may like to take my animals into schools, in order to educate children, as I had done such a good job with him.

That was my eureka! moment, and my life suddenly changed: I had a goal. I haven't looked back since that moment, and now spend every day moving one step closer to the next goal, whatever it may be. It had always been a dream to have a book published, and this one is number two (my first is about nutrition and health).

On the walk home from the nursery, I came up with what became the name of my business – Critterish Allsorts. My then-wife did not like it, but I decided to stick with it. It made me smile then, and still has that effect today, after six years. Customers love it, too! It perfectly describes and sums up the many and varied species that work within the business.

I didn't have any experience of animals in schools, so had no idea of what would be expected of me when I visited, or how I might 'perform.' I began the new venture with birthday parties and summer holiday specials (as the summer holidays had just started), and via the free website I'd built, and my old friend Facebook, the bookings began to arrive. What a wonderful marketing tool social media is!

Gradually, we began to acquire more animals and more bookings. Before long, we were being offered animals that their owners no longer wanted or could care for. A knock at the door one time was answered to a young boy of 6 or 7, standing holding a box, inside of which was a lovely black rabbit. The boy explained that he had been playing in the car park at the local shops, and found the rabbit hopping around. His mother had caught the animal, put it in the box, and told the boy to bring it to us, as she knew that we worked with animals. After taking in the rabbit (who we named Jynx) we put up posters and knocked doors, but nobody claimed her. She's still with us today.

In 2011 my business became an animal assisted therapy provider, thanks to my having a stand at the National Exhibition Centre for the Education Show. Here, I was approached by two women – teachers at a psychiatric hospital – for details of the work I did. I was invited to visit the hospital to try out my services, and I am still visiting every other week now. It was this initial visit that showed me how animals can help people, and instilled in me a passion to do so. Working with the mental health professionals there has allowed me to develop my services and skills into what they are today.

I have added many other customers to the list since then, and work in both private and public sectors, including the NHS. Although others have taken certain exotic creatures (such as guinea pigs) into hospitals before me, I have established myself as a pioneer in animal assisted therapy due to the diverse range of species I work with, with appearances in BBC documentaries and 5 News bulletins, articles in magazines and newspapers around the world, books, and even a few one-hour slots on American radio. Critterish Allsorts is also established as the leading provider of animal assisted therapy services in the UK, and, in early 2017, was voted Best Animal Assisted Therapy Provider for that year. I am very proud to work alongside around fifty animals in what is a thriving business.

My work is my passion, especially when it's with children and adults who suffer from mental illness, however severe. Seeing the effect my animals have on the patients I deal with took me all the way back to my days in the garden with Silky, and I knew, then and there, that this was what I wanted to do always. I have worked towards this objective since, and am happy to say that 98% of the work I do is animal assisted therapy with children and adults who have mental health issues. The remaining 2% involves working in schools with children who have behavioural issues, in care homes, and with the disabled.

The fact that my non-human co-counsellors are rescue animals really helps with the patients, who identify with the animals, and bond with them intensely. As for the disabled, I have animals with disabilities that, again, my clients identify with. It really is miraculous and satisfying work, especially when you see the difference that it makes. Although I regard my animals as co-counsellors, I do not see myself as a counsellor, but rather as a facilitator who organises the work they do alongside medical professionals; delivering the animals' healing to those who need it.

One of the questions I am most often asked is 'How do you train your animals?' and the simple answer is that I *don't* train them. What I do is show each animal endless, unconditional love, compassion, care, support and trust, combined with patience, and they reward me with their trust, unconditional love, and support.

I am completely sure that my animals know exactly what they are doing when they work with me. With each patient, and in different situations, their behaviour varies: for instance, my dog knows the difference between a care home and a psychiatric hospital, and knows when he should be really calm. They receive no reward for acting in a particular way, other than my love and the love of the patients, but they seem quite satisfied with this. Neither do my animals perform tricks: sure, Beanz will give you his paw, but that's not come about from training, it's just something that he began to do.

They are, in effect, medical practitioners and co-counsellors, and I treat them with the respect that this merits. They thrive on it!

And the therapy is not just one-way, either, as the animals benefit from their interaction with the patients (I explain this in the chapters that follow). As previously mentioned, all of my animals are 'rescues,' and I consider myself a rescue also, having lived through a number of life-changing experiences – grief and bereavement, relationship loss and poor health – when my animals have saved me. Most recently I was rescued

Unleashing the healing power of animals

by a butterfly who flew into my life most unexpectedly (subject matter for another book to come in due course!)

At the end of it all, I believe that we are all one, whether human or non-human; regardless of religion or colour, background and upbringing. We were all born from the same sea of life, and we shall all be poured back into it when our time comes.

I hope that you enjoy the biographies of my animals (I do have a few animals who are not rescues, and a chapter at the end of the book provides information about them). There are, as my company name suggests, all sorts of animals for you to meet within these pages: furry ones and scaly ones, and an animal for everyone. My dream and the aim of my business is to see animal assisted therapy become a recognised, mainstream, *prescribed* treatment for mental health conditions, and especially as a first port of call for the treatment of depression and anxiety. I am currently working with doctors and psychologists to establish evidence for why we should be unleashing the healing power of animals.

I also hope that my book may encourage anyone with a passion for both animals and helping others to follow a career path in animal assisted therapy. I receive many enquiries from students and others wishing to change careers and lives about how to become an animal assisted therapy practitioner, and am always happy to assist with these.

I'll leave you with one of my favourite animal quotes –

"What is man without the beasts? If all the beasts were gone, man would die from great loneliness of spirit. For whatever happens to the beasts, soon happens to man. All things are connected."

Chief Sealth (Seattle), Duwamish Tribe, 1850

Visit Hubble and Hattie on the web: www.hubbleandhattie.com
hubbleandhattie.blogspot.co.uk
• Details of all books • Special offers • Newsletter • New book news

2
Beanz – The Border Collie

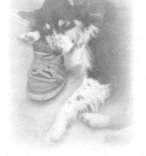

*I was down, I was barely makin' it; she was gone and I couldn't take it;
I was lookin' for a new way of thinkin'; when I'd go to sleep, I'd pray I
wouldn't wake up; well, I want you, I want you to rescue me.*
– Dave Meniketti (Yesterday & Today) *Rescue Me*

It's said that animals choose us rather than the other way around, and I
think that this is very true of animals in need of rescue. A sixth sense, the
most basic of all instincts, seems to guide them toward the person who is
right for them. Have you ever been in the shelter or rescue centre, unsure
of which animal to choose, when one of them wanders over to you? You
pick that one – am I right? Animals are a lot cleverer than we think!

What can I tell you about Beanz? Well, because of my experience
with the family dog when I was young, I am not the biggest lover of dogs.
But Beanz is Beanz; a really special little fellow. Not much is known about
him, other than the fact that he was found on the streets of Eire (southern
Ireland). Nobody knew where he had come from, or his history, and his
age was an estimated 18 months.

Beanz found his way to the Border Collie Trust UK in Colton,
Staffordshire – a very worthwhile charity which visits Ireland once a month
to bring back stray dogs, of which there are a fair few. In Ireland, Collies
are considered working dogs, and if they are not good at their work,
then the attitude seems to be that they are good for nothing. In addition,
Beanz is a tri-colour Collie, which are not well-liked in Ireland.

Beanz did not know what toys were; he had no idea how to play.
He was scared of traffic, to the point where he would fall to the floor and
shake if we were walking along a footpath and traffic passed us. He was
also scared of squeaky toys and loud noises such as shouting and singing.
My ex-wife (let's call her Jean) was instrumental in getting him to walk on a
lead. She was persistent and determined, but most of all she was patient
with him, managing to coax him out on walks; stopping when he needed

to, and reassuring him that he was safe. All credit to her, she got there with him eventually.

One thing that he excelled at, however, was running around in circles, tracking other dogs and children. Get him in an open field with other dogs and he was in his element, running huge sweeping circles around them, and keeping them all within the areas. This gave us the impression that he had done some herding training, although Collies in general do seem to have the herding instinct as part of their make-up.

When Beanz arrived, we already had a dog, a crossbreed and a rescue, who had been left on the doorstep of a veterinary practice when around a week old. She came to us from the veterinary nurse who nursed her and the rest of the litter until they were eight weeks old. Jean had been to the Border Collie rescue, which was local to us, to volunteer her services. Whilst there they asked her to walk a dog, which she was very happy to do: that was why she was there, after all. At home later, Jean recounted how she had walked this dog called Beanz, and how amazing he was. She asked if we could home him.

My immediate response was an emphatic 'No!' We already had a dog, and she was a real handful. I knew, from experience, that Collies are boisterous dogs who require time and effort to care for. We had lots of vivariums – and hence lots of glass – containing snakes and lizards: the potential for disaster and injury to both dog and reptile was huge, and we also had three young children who could get tangled up in the mess. In my mind the risk was too great.

Jean cried and cried, and not just for a few hours, but a few days! Eventually, I thought to myself that I needed to see what was so special about this particular dog, and so, unbeknown to Jean, I visited the rescue centre and asked them if I could walk Beanz, having explained about Jean's earlier visit and encounter with him.

Beanz was made ready and I was handed his lead. He gave me this happy look (I mean he was really smiling) – obviously out to impress – that asked 'Where are we going?' We set off and I talked to Beanz as we walked. I asked him all sorts of questions – what it was that Jean had found so special about him; where he had come from; what had happened to him, etc.

Stopping at about middle-distance (Beanz wanted to keep going), we sat down on the grass. I was stroking him and talking to him, and Beanz was looking at me with that smile and those eyes, apparently listening intently to what I was saying. "You know something?" I asked him. He smiled. "There *is* something really special about you. I wonder if the rescue would allow us to take you home to see how you get on? Only a trial, though, you understand." I explained to him about the vivariums, and the mad dog who already shared our home, as I walked him back to the office.

Explaining our home situation I asked if Beanz could have a trial day at our home, to see how he was around the other animals. It wasn't something that the rescue normally did, but, given the circumstances, it was felt that this was a good idea.

Once home Beanz was brilliant. Gentle and respectful indoors, outside he was a proper dog. Perfect behaviour that hasn't changed. He had to go back to the rescue for a week to be neutered, and since then he has gone from strength to strength. We have found out much about him, but, you know, he hasn't barked once in all the years he has been with us, and we have no idea what happened to his bark.

Jean and I parted in 2014, by which time we had acquired a third dog. When she left, she took two of the dogs, but left Beanz. She didn't abandon him, it's just that she realised Beanz and I had become a pair, a partnership, and he was more my dog than hers, especially given our working relationship. It's something I shall be forever grateful to her for.

Beanz, on the other hand, was heartbroken by the loss of his group (as was I), and especially the two dogs he shared his space with, and it took him a good while to get over this. His behaviour took a step backwards in terms of toileting indoors; he was unhappy in himself – his smile disappeared for a while – and he was (for want of a better word) depressed ... but then we both were. We supported each other and came out of it together. Other potential group members came and went until, eventually, everything settled and a 'butterfly' flew into our lives which resulted in a smaller group, but one that was less fragile and more 'together.' Beanz loves children, and is especially happy when my partner's niece visits us.

Watching a TV show in which celebrities attempted to work with Collies in order to move sheep around a series of obstacles, I noticed that Beanz was responding to the commands, inasmuch as he was moving his ears when they were voiced. I noted down the commands to try out with Beanz the next day. It was amazing: he seemed to understand them all – 'come by,' 'lie down,' 'wait,' 'walk.' I had him running after a ball and rounding it up at the same time. Amazing dog. It confirmed what I already suspected: Beanz had been a working dog at some point.

I think when it comes to rescuing a dog – any animal, in fact – you have to work out what has formed them in order to move forward. It was obvious to us that Beanz had been out on the street for a while, had had bad experiences with traffic, squeaky toys (possibly used for 'training' or 'discipline'), and other things, and we now figured that he had been a working dog at some point.

Discovering what drives an animal, and gives them the best feeling of happiness and security (a nice blanket to lie on, kindness, lots of love and attention (at least in the early days), a need to be close to you always), is key, and the rewards are fantastic. Important for a rescue animal is a sense of security, and a high level of emotional support, to help them feel 'normal' again.

Unleashing the healing power of animals

What motivates Beanz? Freedom, shelter, play, learning, and his work – he loves it, seriously loves it. From the moment I put on my work shirt he thrives on it. When we arrive at our destination, he knows where we are and exactly how to behave. For instance, he behaves differently in a care home or dementia ward to how he would in a psychiatric hospital situation with younger, more active people, and differently again in a critical care unit. He knows which patients want to pet him and talk to him, and he knows which want to play with him and have some fun. All of this he has intuitively learned, without any help from me, from his time as a therapy animal. That dog just smiles all day long, and I have never seen him happier than when he is working. He always does me really proud, and has never let me down.

And what does a typical day involve for Beanz? He doesn't mind being around the house, but is happiest when he's doing something. He seems to get so much more from his work. It's therapy for him, too!

Wherever we are working I do not travel for longer than two hours with any of my animals, as it is not fair on them to be cooped up in a car for hours on end. Even then, we stop for a rest break at some point so that I can check on them, and allow Beanz to get out of the car and stretch his legs, and do anything else he needs to. Whilst driving I talk to the animals, especially Beanz (who normally travels in the back), as I figure that he gets reassurance from hearing my voice and knowing I am there.

Arriving at our destination Beanz's face lights up, and he gets so excited! He recognises those places we regularly visit, but then all dogs do that – on walks, in particular. An interesting fact I discovered a few years ago is that a dog's sense of smell is so attuned to their surroundings that they can work out short cuts to and from their destination! Impressive!

Entering the venue, Beanz can tell by the smell what sort of place it is, even though I cannot smell a tangible difference. His tail is always in the air, swinging gently side to side, his eyes wide in anticipation, his tongue lolling from his mouth; his expression happy and excited. We will then be escorted onto a ward or into a room where patients will visit us. Some just want to sit with Beanz and stroke him, and others want to play.

In a session the animal dictates what happens, and if they have had enough or no longer want to interact with a patient, then they are not forced to do so. Likewise, if an animal no longer wants to take part in a session then the session ends. The professionals I work with respect this, as do the patients, although it can be hard for them to accept sometimes as there is inevitably a feeling of rejection. In this instance, explaining that it is no different to them deciding that they no longer wish to take part in a session helps them to understand that Beanz is not rejecting them.

Beanz gets a comfort break between each session, in which he can run around an open area outside and do what he needs to. Sessions can involve him playing with a ball, or simply sitting and being petted; sometimes a session will involve going out into the community with

BEANZ PLAYS BALL

I've already mentioned that when Beanz arrived with us he did not understand play: well, the following is the story of how Beanz learnt to play, which also demonstrates how his work is also therapeutic for him.

We used to visit a psychiatric hospital in the north of England, where the majority of patients were severely autistic (amongst other things). The patients were really keen for Beanz to play, because, in their eyes, that's what dogs do! They would therefore spend hour upon hour throwing a ball for him, or trying to teach him tricks – they were very persistent. For almost twelve months they threw Beanz the ball, telling him to 'fetch,' but he simply looked at them with his tongue hanging out the side of his mouth.

I tried telling them that they would not get him to bring the ball: after all, I had tried every day for six months to get him to do this, without success. Anyway, after about ten months (that's around twenty day-long visits) of Beanz watching the patients throwing the toy for him, but then fetching it themselves, one day, as the ball was thrown, Beanz followed its trajectory through the air with his eyes ... then his legs ... picked it up, and brought it to me. I immediately began to cry at seeing Beanz play, and it remains one of my most beautiful memories of our time together. If it wasn't for the guys in that hospital, I'm not sure that Beanz would be playing with toys even now. Oh, and you should have seen his little face, he was so proud of himself. And who could blame him?

After that Beanz was like a child with a new toy (which I suppose he was); he could not get enough. He would bring the ball and drop it at just about anyone's feet. Playing gave Beanz a completely new lease of life, a whole new dimension; he was like a puppy again. So you see, although he was the therapy dog, his work and, in particular, those patients, had, unwittingly, been his therapy, too. They taught him how to play, and enhanced his life. Neither Beanz or I will ever be able to thank them enough for that.

Animal assisted therapy is a two-way street. With a rescue animal it teaches them that it is possible for humans to love and treat them right regardless of their background, and it teaches them that they can trust again. With the patients it lets them see them that they are worthy of love and trust, and helps bring down barriers that may have been blocking this understanding.

Unleashing the healing power of animals

an individual for a walk. People love to walk dogs! Walking a dog is a sociable activity that brings with it many aspects, such as acceptance (being part of the community as we pass others walking their dogs), and interaction (acknowledging others and greeting them, which, in itself, is enough to bestow a feeling of belonging on someone unused to being part of a community). Sometimes, even a conversation about the dog(s) will develop as a result, which teaches much about interacting in an acceptable way in the outside world; it also means that the focus of the conversation is not on the patient, for a change, but on the dog, and is therefore less threatening.

Dog walking is particularly useful when a patient is being rehabilitated into the local community, and also allows the professionals to assess, in some part, an individual's ability to behave appropriately within the community.

A dog in therapy sessions can also help in many other ways. There are the obvious benefits of furry animals in therapy, inasmuch as stroking them releases the feel good hormones oxytocin and serotonin into the body, as well as the feeling of calmness that results from a reduced heart rate.

We worked with Virgin Trains on a few occasions, where we carried out an experiment with commuters. Setting up with several animals in the station concourse, commuters were offered the opportunity to spend a few minutes at the end of their journey, simply sitting with an animal. Commuting can be a stressful experience, and the idea behind this experiment was that spending a few minutes in the calming company of an animal might help restore the natural balance of endorphins, and lead to a safer and more pleasurable onward journey home. On one of these occasions, we were accompanied by a PhD student from the University of Central Lancashire who took 'before and after' blood pressure and heart rate readings of those who participated. The results showed that 95% of the commuters measured had reduced blood pressure and heart rate readings. Although it was only a small sample of people (about 20) the beneficial results were clear to see.

A less obvious benefit is the knowledge individuals gain from interacting with me and my animals, such as how much financial cost and effort is involved in caring for them, which allows an individual to make an informed decision about whether or not a particular creature would make a good companion animal for them, once they are rehabilitated. The beauty of working with rescue animals is that it encourages individuals to want to rehome a rescue animal, rather than buy from a breeder, which is great news for all the animals waiting patiently for their forever home.

Beanz also teaches individuals about the importance of grooming. I am often asked which of my animals is the hardest to look after, and my answer is always Beanz. People are generally surprised by this, but once I have explained the requirements of looking after a dog, they soon understand. Dogs need regular grooming (and especially long-haired animals like Beanz), otherwise they can develop knots in their hair, leading to matting, which can be painful and result in skin disease.

I've used the term 'patients' a lot in this chapter, which is because the majority of work that I do with Beanz and my other animals is within psychiatric hospitals, although we also work in care homes, special schools, and similar organisations.

Of course, dogs are not a favourite with everyone. We live in a multicultural, multi-society world, where, for example, some religions forbid interaction with dogs, as they are regarded as unclean. This is one reason why I began using a multitude of different species in my work. In addition, some people are allergic to fur and hair, and, with the increase in reptile ownership, some prefer animals of a more exotic nature.

The following chapters explore some of the species of animal I work with, and explain how they have a therapeutic effect on the individuals I treat. For example, I was approached by the mother of a 10-year-old girl, Caitlin. Caitlin was afraid of dogs – a condition known as cynophobia – which caused problems for the family wherever they went: even the smallest trip was difficult. A journey to school would take longer than it should, as an encounter with a dog would cause Caitlin to freeze, grab hold of her mom's arm, and hide behind her. Wherever they went, between them, they would do a running commentary whilst surveying the area – arrival in a park car park, for instance, would initiate the commentary: how many of the cars contained dogs?; what sort of dogs were they?; etc. It really was a struggle for the whole family.

Beanz's temperament makes him perfect for dealing with a problem like this; his gentle nature really helps. Beanz obviously had no idea about Caitlin's problem: he just wants to play! Caitlin is a keen footballer herself, so this gave the two something in common from the outset and we would meet Caitlin, initially every week, at a local park, and spend an hour playing with Beanz and interacting with him (stroking, feeding him treats, talking to him, giving him cues, and walking him on a lead) in controlled and supervised conditions.

Caitlin became more and more confident around Beanz as the weeks went on, but shied away from other dogs we encountered. We would talk about them as they approached, and whilst Caitlin either hid behind her mom or completely avoided the dog, preferring to stay in the company of Beanz, her mom and I would pet the other dog, to encourage Caitlin to do the same. In time, Caitlin became more and more confident; not just with Beanz, but with dogs in general. Controlled exposure like this gradually habituated Caitlin, firstly to Beanz, and then to dogs in general, allowing her confidence to grow.

We had a few significant breakthroughs. Walks to school became less fraught, with a calmer reaction to dogs she encountered. For the first time, Caitlin was able to visit friends and relatives with dogs, going into their homes and being in the presence of their dogs. A family holiday in Perranporth, Cornwall (where the family has a holiday home, and regularly visits) would normally be a tense affair, especially on the local beach where there would usually be a number of dogs. With Beanz's help, and the regular interactions that Caitlin was having with Beanz and other dogs we encountered, the family was able to spend relaxed family time on the beach in the company of dogs for the first time.

Beanz helped change this family's entire dynamic, by helping Caitlin to overcome her cynophobia. It's not clear where Caitlin's irrational fear of dogs came from, but this condition is a lot more common than we may realise. This is where other animals come into play in a therapy situation, and the more variety on offer, the more people can be treated and helped. That said, not all creatures will make good therapy animals, because of their natural behaviours and temperaments, and these aspects should be assessed and considered when choosing an animal for therapy.

Beanz and I continue our work with Caitlin, but much less frequently now as her confidence with dogs has grown so much. It has been truly beautiful to see Caitlin's relationship with dogs blossom – and with Beanz in particular – and her confidence grow so much. One of the reasons that Beanz and I continue to see Caitlin is because of the lovely relationship that the two of them enjoy. There are plans to take Beanz to agility classes in the future, and for Caitlin to be involved in that in some way. The therapy continues with each interaction, but becomes more and more subtle each time, until it will eventually no longer be needed. A real therapy success!

By just being himself, Beanz has also helped others who did not like dogs – for religious reasons or otherwise – to appreciate his species, and appreciate that they are neither dirty or vicious animals. This can only be good news for both dogs and people.

A final paragraph about Beanz's own continuing development and confidence-building.

In March 2014, just a few years after arriving with us, Beanz had his acting debut, playing Sandy in a local production of the musical *Annie*. Once again, Beanz thrived, not only on the attention he received, but also the challenge of what he had to do. There were no lines to learn, of course, but he did have to move around the stage amongst other characters. His tail did not stop wagging the entire time, and neither did his winning smile leave his face. Beanz more than rose to the occasion, and not only did he learn his moves, he also learnt his cues, knowing, by what the other actors said, when he should move and to where.

Each night he would take the last bow, and get the largest cheer and round of applause, and rightly so. Beanz really *is* a star!

Sebastian – The Chinchilla
3

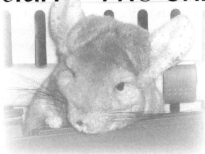

Sebastian is a Chinchilla, a soft, grey, rodent-type animal from South America. When I talk about Sebastian with children, we describe him as a cross between a mouse and a squirrel. Indeed, one could be forgiven for imagining he is the mouse in the wonderful book *The Gruffalo* – still one of my favourite children's books of all time!

Sebastian was rescued from a Chinchilla breeder. Though Chinchillas do not necessarily mate for life, if they are paired they can establish a very close bond, and refuse to mate with other Chinchillas. This was the case with Sebastian, and why the breeder no longer wanted him, as he was no longer of any use for breeding. Which is where we came in, when he was four years old.

Sebastian has come a long way since then: from a Chinchilla who did not like to be touched, to a therapy animal who thrives on being the centre of attention. He is one of the most popular animals I work with, and always tops the favourite lists of patients, young and old.

Why he is so popular, and how he came to be so tame, is a question I get asked quite often. As I've already said, I do not train any of my animals. I do not use clickers or treats to persuade them to do things; they do what they do from free will because they are happy to do so, and in fact appear to relish their work. If, at any time, this changes, the animal concerned is taken out of service and reassessed, which may mean that he or she is retired from their work as a therapy animal, and spends the rest of their life as my pet.

When we collected Sebastian from his owner he was a breeding animal. Breeding animals are not pets; nor are they treated as such, and, when rescuing an animal, this is certainly something to consider. An ex-breeding animal will require a lot of attention from you as their new companion because they will not have received the attention that a companion animal usually will have. They will generally have been permanently confined to a cage, and simply fed, watered, cleaned, and encouraged to breed as often as possible. (We have more than one ex- breeding animal at Critterish Cottage, and I talk about these in a later chapter.)

I had to decide on a course of action with Sebastian, and my initial plan was not to ask him to be a therapy animal, but just to show him that he was loved, and that he could trust me, so that he could be a pet for my family, and enjoy interaction with his human companions.

How was this achieved? Slowly and steadily, is how! Chinchillas are notoriously flighty animals – they simply do not sit still. After his arrival, I had let Sebastian have a run around the lounge, and he was everywhere – behind the TV nibbling on cables, on the sofa, etc. The first challenge, therefore, was to get Sebastian to stay still long enough to sniff my finger through the bars of his enclosure.

I discovered that Sebastian tended to sit still when I opened his cage to feed him – food is a great motivator for animals – so each day when I fed him, I left my hand by the bowl. He would approach but stop short of his bowl, nervous of my hand. After a few days of this, he became used to my hand being there, and this was the first time that he and I had a physical connection of his choosing, although he would still run away after sniffing my hand (we found that putting fingers through bars for him to sniff resulted in said fingers getting bitten!).

The next step was to stroke him. Now, I had felt Sebastian's fur before (when I had to catch him in the lounge), and it was luxuriously soft. Chinchillas have around 50-100 hairs per follicle, meaning that their fur is very soft and dense, which is what made it so desirable to furriers in the early to mid-1900s. It was in the mid-16th century that Chinchilla fur was first sent to Europe, but it was not until the late 19th century that Chinchilla fur became as popular as it did. It was possible to feed a family for a month from the sale of just one pelt, if a Chinchilla could be found! They are nocturnal; elusive and quick in the wild where they live, high up in the Andes Mountains. In 1910, those states in the Chinchilla's locale united to ban the trade in the animal's fur, though feared they were too late and that extinction was inevitable.

Salvation came in the most unlikely guise – fur farming. In 1923, one Mathias Chapman obtained permission from Chile to trap eleven animals for breeding, which took him three years to do (told you they were tricky to catch!). Chapman initially intended to breed the animals for pets, but changed his mind, and began farming them for fur. There are Chinchilla farms in the Americas and Europe today, and all of their stock are thought to be descended from Chapman's original eleven animals. Fur farming diverted demand from the wild Chinchilla population, and allowed it to increase in number, although the Chinchilla still is regarded as critically endangered by the International Union for Conservation of Nature. It's a great shame that extinction was only avoided because of legalised fur farming, but it is something, at least.

Sebastian – The Chinchilla

Some interesting facts there about Sebastian and his clan, but, yes, Chinchilla fur is probably the softest you will ever feel. When I look at the faces of patients who handle Sebastian for the first time, it's easy to understand why the little fella is so popular.

It was a while before Sebastian felt sufficiently at ease with me that I was able to feel his luxurious fur myself, but, leaving my hand by his bowl in the hope that, one day, he may do more than sniff it, eventually paid off, when he allowed me to stroke him on his terms. This was a truly beautiful day, and a great reward for our patience.

We continued like this for a long time, until he was allowing me to stroke his head and his back, though was very guarded about having his tail touched. This was understandable, as Chinchillas use their tails for balance, and it is therefore a particularly sensitive part of their body.

In time, Sebastian would climb out of his cage to be with the family, running around on the sofa and across laps. We were all talking to Sebastian whenever we were close to his cage, and had introduced ourselves to him, so he had become used to us. He seemed happy hopping around and sharing himself between us all. He was getting used to people at last. This was huge for Sebastian and for us: a true turning point. Experiencing the joy that he gave us made me want to share it with others. I decided to see how he was with people he didn't know ...

I waited for Sebastian to become used to his transport box on his terms: smelling it and exploring; gradually finding his way inside where towels embroidered with the company logo provided something comfortable for him to sit on, and, if he wanted to, turn into a 'nest.' A comfortable animal is a happy animal, and a happy animal is one who will respond positively during interaction.

Once he was used to his box, it was time to go out with him. At this juncture, Sebastian was nice and calm when handled – it's unusual for a Chinchilla to simply sit on one's hand and not move, but Sebastian would happily do so, allowing himself to be stroked.

His first therapy visit was to a care home, and, from the moment I got him out of his box, and the residents greeted him with a resounding 'aaahhhhh,' I knew he was going to be a hit. The residents loved him and his soft fur – 'luxurious' was the word they used to describe him. Many of the residents were of an age to remember when Chinchilla fur was in vogue, and a couple even commented that their mother had a coat or stole made from Chinchilla fur.

Sebastian sat patiently on my hand as I told the residents his story, and a little about Chinchillas in general, and continued to sit as we walked around the room chatting to everyone. He allowed himself to be stroked without any sign of nervousness or fear ... which was when I realised that Sebastian really and truly trusted me, and felt like he belonged.

One of the residents asked if she could hold him: I wasn't sure, but, right on cue, Sebastian hopped off my hand and onto the lady's lap!

Unleashing the healing power of animals

He had made up his own mind.

Over the next few months, Sebastian became more and more accustomed to what we did during our visits, and began to enjoy it more and more. One day he hopped up onto my shoulder from my hand, to the delight of the people in the room. He sat there, tickling my neck with his whiskers: it felt so nice, as if he wanted to be close to me. His self-assurance increased, and he became more and more confident in his own skin, sharing himself between chairs and patients, or residents, depending on where we were.

Sebastian is around ten years old now (Chinchillas are surprisingly long-lived to around 18 or 20 years) and, over the last five or six years, he has become one of the most confident, happy, and popular animals I have had the pleasure of sharing my life and work with. He seems to know that I will only ever do my best for him, and rewards me with his trust.

More recently, Sebastian demonstrated the work he does when he joined me on a careers talk at a local primary school. One of the pupils – Caitlin, who featured in the last chapter – was trying to find a way to deal with her fear of dogs, and came across our website. The next day she passed the details to her head teacher, who was interested in our work, and invited us to talk to Year 6 pupils about what we did.

Five of the pupils sat in a row, and Sebastian sat in the lap of the first. After that pupil had given him a fuss, he moved on to the next, and so on, until he had been with each of them. He did this of his own volition, and in his own time, moving from one to the next, stopping for a fuss, and then continuing on his way.

Sebastian appears to love his work, and is very comfortable with what he does, thriving in every situation. He has a special effect on people: calming and reassuring, but also exhilarating at the same time. The feel of his fur is particularly reassuring, I have found, especially to teenagers, who just want to cuddle him and hold him close. I think the reason for this is that Sebastian is soft, with really thick fur ... and about the size of a teddy bear! Teenagers, especially teenage girls, are at a stage in their lives when the security and comfort of a teddy bear is a recent (and maybe even current) memory, and anyone feeling vulnerable is even more receptive to Sebastian's teddy bear charms! Holding him in their hands or on their lap seems to have a familiar, reassuring quality that makes them feel safe and secure.

The exhilaration comes when Sebastian begins to move around! He hops and he jumps, his little feet making the most delightful noises as he scurries back and forth sharing himself between people. His movements and the sound of his feet are amusing. He will stop, sit up, and look around, holding up his front paws, occasionally brushing his nose with one of them, making everyone melt with adoration for him. An animal demonstrating natural behaviours right in front of them – one with the freedom to just 'be' – is an amazing thing to behold for anyone, but especially those people who do not have companion animals in their current situation.

The therapeutic benefits that improve the wellbeing of all extend even to the staff: for themselves, but also by witnessing the people they care for in a completely different light. This can positively impact the interaction between residents and carers going both ways, the overall result of which is an improvement in relationships within the unit, and a calmer environment.

Finally (I almost forgot!), I need to tell you about the girl next door: Lulu, a very pretty female Chinchilla. Now, I don't want baby Chinchillas arriving on the scene – cute as they may be. My view is that the already-too-many animals in rescue centres should find love and a home of their own before any more are purchased from breeders, so Lulu lives in the cage next door to Sebastian, and they rub noses between the bars, and 'talk' to each other. Another interesting fact about Chinchillas is that they 'bark' as a way of communicating (imagine the noise a Yorkshire Terrier on helium might make): it's a very strange sound, and quite disconcerting when heard for the first time at 3am!

Lulu is another rescue Chinchilla, about a year Sebastian's junior, who lived with a family. Lulu became pregnant and gave birth at around the same time as the lady of the house did. Human babies, of course, demand a lot of time and attention, which meant that Lulu did not get the time and attention that her owner felt she needed and deserved. Quite rightly, therefore, she decided that Lulu and her son should be re-homed, and we took them both.

Lulu had not been handled for almost two years, and was therefore almost wild in her instincts – as we all know, animals left to their own devices often become feral, reverting to their wild behaviours. Despite being regularly fed and cleaned, and having a degree of human contact, Lulu had done just that.

I am working with her, as I did with Sebastian, to try and gain her trust, and my partner, Kat, has also been hugely influential in this area – in fact, Lulu responds more to Kat than to me; they have a real connection. It has taken four years to reach this stage, and she will only allow me to tickle her between her ears since Kat began to interact with her. She does respond very much to sounds, and seems to enjoy it when we speak to her. She knows her name and responds to our voices, and will accept a certain level of interaction, but nothing like Sebastian. Why this is I do not know, but patience and perseverance are my watchwords. I want her to enjoy being a companion animal first and foremost, and not feel nervous of human company.

For the time being Lulu is able to be close to another of her kind, and I think that she finds this reassuring. They can smell each other, they can see each other, they can 'talk' to each other, and both seem happy. When Sebastian returns home from work with me, the first thing he does when back in his enclosure is go to the bars and check on Lulu. It's lovely to see, and we are pleased that they enjoy each other's company.

LOSING LULU

During the writing of this book, Sebastian's friend, Lulu, passed away. This event was traumatic for the little Chinchilla, who was distraught by the loss of his mate. One of the reactions to stress in Chinchillas is chewing of the tail, a body part that they use for balance, and therefore vital to his well-being. Chinchillas are nocturnal; Lulu's demise occurred during the night, which is when Sebastian began to 'self-harm.'

When I went in to see the animals that morning, I found not only that Lulu had died, but that Sebastian had a chunk missing out of his tail, where he had been chewing it. Obviously, the wound was treated, but I also treated the grief that Sebastian was experiencing. I altered his enclosure so that the bottom part was enclosed to give him privacy, and also devoted a lot of my time and energy to helping him through his grief.

The wound has healed nicely and Sebastian is back to his usual happy self, although he is a lot closer to me as a result of what happened. 'Out of all negatives, there comes a positive,' and the positive in this case is that Sebastian is now able to help people with a specific mental health issue – those who self-harm – that he wasn't able to previously.

I recently began seeing a teenager with mental health issues, one of which is that she self-harms. Sebastian's first meeting with her demonstrated his new-found ability, as the first thing that this young person saw was the scar on the Chinchilla's tail.

"What happened to his tail?" she asked, and, as I told her the story, her face softened, as she obviously identified with what Sebastian had done. Not only that, but she also understood Sebastian's motivation. I was with a psychologist at the time, and we decided to explore this reaction further.

We asked the patient how she thought Sebastian had felt whilst self-harming, and how she thought I may have felt when I discovered what he'd done. Speaking as if from Sebastian's viewpoint, the young girl was actually talking for the very first time about her own emotions and motivation, the consequences of her actions for her parents, and their feelings about it.

The psychologist was astounded that an animal could have such an impact on somebody with a mental illness, and it reaffirmed his belief in animals as a therapeutic medium. The patient was able to feel more comfortable talking about her problem and associated emotions, as well as draw comfort from knowing she was not alone, and that, by addressing the problem, there was light at the end of the tunnel – a light that Sebastian had found.

After this initial session, Sebastian was requested by this particular patient for each of her regular sessions. Through their common issue of self-harming they had formed a bond, a bond that led to the patient wanting to help Sebastian continue to get better, at the same time as he was helping her to do the same.

This benefit has also been demonstrated in other recent sessions within a CAMHS (Child & Adolescent Mental Health Services) unit that I visit, where patients have noticed Sebastian's tail, and asked the same question. The answer has always led to a discussion about self-harm, be this a simple conclusion of "Well, if he can get through it then so can I," or a more in-depth exploration of cause and consequence. Either way, the outcome is always a positive one for the patient in terms of dealing with their mental health issue.

4
Mooch – The Monitor Lizard

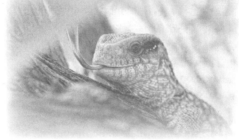

Mooch was one hell of an animal. A lizard, a Savannah or Bosc Monitor Lizard – one of those *big* lizards with a huge, blue, forked tongue. He had a very special spirit: kind and gentle, that you could see in his eyes.

Sadly, Mooch passed away after almost 12 months with us: his story was short but sweet, and I am so glad that we had time together. He gave me nearly twelve very happy months, and I think about him every single day, because we had such a very special relationship.

When I am unhappy or have problems, I still talk to him. I appreciate how that may sound, but I feel him all around me all of the time, giving me strength. I am pretty sure, dear reader, that you, too, have felt this strength from a departed animal; especially one with whom you had a particularly deep connection.

As big and scary-looking as he was, Mooch was a gentle giant who wowed everybody he met. In terms of our relationship, every single person who saw us together recognised the special bond we had. He was also comfortable around other animals, and could be trusted with them. His vivarium would be left open and he would come and go as he pleased, wandering around the house, sleeping with the cats, and climbing the stairs to find me for a cuddle.

I have some very fond memories of our time together. I even went as far as to have a tattoo of Mooch on my right shoulder, just after he died. It is a picture of his face, taken from a professional photograph by a friend of mine.

For those of you of a spiritual nature like me, three days before Mooch departed this earthly plane, the last photographs of him were taken at a children's party. The photographs clearly show 'orbs' (thought to be globes of energy moving from one place to another) bouncing about all over the hall, but only when Mooch was in the photograph: those which did not feature Mooch did not have the orbs. In one photo an orb is resting on top of Mooch's travel box, with him inside it. To me, this is confirmation that animals are not only sentient beings, as we are, but that they also have spirits, as we do. This reinforces my belief that we are all one with each other and with nature – a cup of water taken from the lake of life, a lake that we are poured back into when we die, to be given life once more. My beliefs, of course, and not those that everyone will subscribe to.

Many people believe that orbs are particles of dust or moisture reflecting light, and, in some cases, this is a very plausible explanation. In this case, however, they only appeared in those photographs in which Mooch appeared ...

When I decide on a name for the animals with whom I share my life, I like to observe them for a while to find a name that suits their personality. Mooch was so-named because he liked to walk around exploring, but with no real purpose.

Obviously, I had no idea of what his life had been like before we met, and that day was a real eye-opener. Life had apparently not been good for Mooch, as he had lived in a house with people who had no idea how to care for him. One of the problems we find when rescuing exotic animals is that sometimes those who want to keep them as pets have no idea about what's involved. Those who sell reptiles are also partly to blame, as they do not ask the right questions to ensure that the purchaser has done their research. Eventually, the owner finds caring for their reptile just too much, and we end up with a totally unhappy situation where the animal is either abandoned in the wild to fend for themselves (as you will read in later chapters), or poorly cared for with resultant health and well-being issues, which was Mooch's predicament. Baby Monitor Lizards are small and extremely cute, but people often have no idea of how big they grow, or what they need in order to lead a happy life.

Mooch was being kept in a dark cupboard with no natural light. UVB (ultra violet B) light is responsible for the production of vitamin D3, which is necessary for any animal's health and development. All diurnal (active during the day) and crepuscular (active at twilight) reptiles should have 10 to 12 hours' exposure daily, and if access to natural sunlight is not possible it is essential that special UVB lamps/strip-lights are made available to a lizard.

There was also no heat source in the cupboard. Reptiles cannot generate their own heat so this is essential not only for warmth but for proper digestion of food. A lot of this explains why Mooch enjoyed his new-found freedom so much, when we were able to give it to him.

Mooch's diet had consisted of dog food, which is not a suitable food for *any* lizard, but especially his type. In the wild, Monitor Lizards eat a varied diet of insects, eggs, small mammals, and viscera. Dog food is high in protein that can cause a lizard to become obese and deficient in vitamins. Feeding a proper diet is essential. It was clear from the start that Mooch would require special dietary attention – and he got it.

Unleashing the healing power of animals

Mooch's previous owners had obviously taken on too much when they decided to buy a Monitor Lizard. They told me when I went to collect him that he was a 'cute baby' when they bought him, who they thought would not grow any bigger. This is where pet shop staff should be asking questions, and explaining that lizards like Mooch are not for the beginner, especially considering their specialised dietary and habitat requirements. They should also explain what size the animal will grow to – and that they will do so very quickly! Mooch's species can reach a size of three feet and get quite heavy: other types of Monitor Lizard can grow even bigger! Another important point is that if the animals are not given the time and attention they need, they can become quite aggressive, and defensive of their space.

Also in the house that Mooch was taken from were other poor animals who were not being properly cared for. The dead Tarantula in a box on the window sill was assumed to be 'ill' – I put them right on that one! Also in the same room as Mooch's cupboard was a rabbit in a hamster cage. The cage was barely big enough for the rabbit, and the poor thing could not even turn around. I offered to take the rabbit, too, but they refused, so I had no choice but to call in the RSPCA.

That was Mooch's previous life, and the life that he was leaving behind for good, because as soon as I saw Mooch and the conditions he was being kept in, I was in no doubt that he was coming home with me. I put him into a transport box and carried him out of the house and into a car as quickly as I could. Both me and my stepdaughter who was with me were upset about the conditions that animals were being kept in in that house.

It was summertime when I collected Mooch – warm and bright; the sun shining – and, despite the fact that we had quite a long drive, I knew that it would still be light when we arrived home. As far as I was aware, Mooch had never seen the sun, let alone felt it; had never experienced the outside, or the breeze on his skin. I really did feel for him and what he had missed for so long, so the first thing we did when we got home was to give Mooch time outside in the garden, in the sun, and watched, whilst he stretched his legs and explored. My three stepchildren were playing in the evening sun, and watching the new addition to our family as we tried to come up with a name for him.

Mooch did not appear at all bothered by what was going on around him, and seemed more interested in soaking up what heat he could from the sun, and meeting the other animals in the garden. His amazing tongue flicked in and out, taking in all of the new smells – grass, flowers, earth, trees – and listening to birds singing; children laughing. I tried to put myself in his shoes, experiencing all of this for the very first time. It must have been amazing!

Mooch seemed happy with his freedom, and did not try to run or get away, and neither was he even mildly aggressive. Rescue animals seem to realise that they are in a better place, and are grateful to be there.

The other animals in the garden were rabbits and guinea pigs, and Joseph the rabbit was the first that Mooch met. Joseph was also the first animal to join our household, three years previously, and he had an extremely happy and calm disposition – a great therapy animal. Their encounter was captured on camera. Mooch was extremely interested in Joseph in a good way, and the rabbit did not once react negatively, seeming to greet each other with mutual respect. It was good to see, and I knew from that moment that Mooch was going to make a great therapy animal.

Mooch wandered about the garden, digging in the dirt searching for bugs, meeting the other animals, and even climbing trees! It was fabulous to see just how happy he was.

I had organised a nice new home for Mooch, a vivarium that contained places to dig and things to climb, and which allowed me to hide food for him to find. He seemed to prefer being outside the vivarium, though, which is understandable, so he was given free run of the house, and only used his vivarium for sleeping and toileting (no matter where he was, he would always go back to his vivarium to toilet). The other animals free-roaming in the house were five cats and a dog, and Mooch could often be found sleeping or resting with the cats, who would stretch out on the underfloor heating. Live food – locusts – were served on the floor of the front room or kitchen. He also loved taking a bath, which was great for his muscle tone as he would be required to swim. We had many fun times with Mooch, and would take him walking on a lead and harness, around the neighbourhood and at various events. This activity was also particularly popular with the psychiatric patients that he visited. He frequently sought out my lap on which to sleep, as if he just wanted to be with me.

Everybody who saw us together commented on how close we were. I liked being with Mooch: it just felt right. Our relationship was second to none, and something I've not experienced with another animal, not even my first rabbit all those years ago. We spent every moment we could in each other's company, and my reward for this was an animal who trusted me totally, not only to handle him, but also when it came to working with other people – patients in psychiatric hospitals and other clients. He seemed to have so much positive energy to give, and he would give it 100% whenever he was asked to. Being with Mooch was just amazing, wherever we were. He was a magnificent, majestic creature: I was proud to be with him, and proud that he was my friend.

As well as working we spent time together playing and cuddling. I would hold Mooch against my shoulder, and talk to him, tickling the soft spots on the sides of his neck. He would rest his head on my shoulder, taking in the smells and heat from my body, no doubt. I could feel his love for me radiating from him, we had something really special, which I think was instrumental in how my relationship with nature and other animals developed. All animals appreciate love and patience.

Mooch was very popular in therapy sessions, especially with children and younger adults. In psychiatric hospitals, the patients liked to see how he moved and how he behaved, and also liked to walk him around the gardens on his lead. On occasion he would sit with a patient and just allow himself to be stroked. Each animal is an individual, and patients identified with Mooch for unique reasons. It's quite possible – likely, even – that many of those we worked with felt his pain, having experienced similar emotions themselves. They felt an immediate link, a compassion, that brought out a protective side in them that not even their carers had witnessed.

Mooch helped many of the psychiatric patients we visited overcome the fears they had. By explaining everything about him, and demonstrating his gentle nature, patients soon picked up on his positive vibes, which seemed to transfer to them. This positivity and allaying of fears manifested itself in their increased self-esteem, in turn leading to increased confidence and well-being.

Mooch was able to fulfil two particular roles known to promote the release of feel good hormones in the brain: he could be stroked like a cat, and walked like a dog. Most importantly, patients were able to witness him being a lizard. Although domesticated to a point, unlike the usual domesticated animals lizards retain their primal, wild instincts, so when left to roam a large area of hospital courtyard planted with shrubs, it was both fun and interesting to watch him perform natural behaviours.

Sadly, though, all good things must come to an end, and, although it had not been apparent, Mooch was not well. Reptiles can hide illness quite well, much like birds of prey can, and so everything had appeared to be as it should: he was eating, he was active, and he seemed his usual self.

Mooch's last event was a little girl's birthday party, where it was great to see him enjoying himself. We had a routine whereby guests would guess the different aspects of Mooch's life in the wild, and I would elaborate on these, showing them how he moved, and how he could climb up and down trees. The gasps when he was taken from his box were always loud and excited, but with a hint of nervous energy. I liked the effect he had on people, he was truly a magnificent critter who was totally deserving of the awe and wonder he generated. Kids rarely get to experience animals such as Mooch, and often do not even know they exist, so he was doing a great PR job for reptiles in particular, and animals in general.

We finished the party that Sunday, and everything seemed normal, the only exception being that Mooch had not had his usual poo in his carriage box. I didn't think too much of it, but decided to keep my eye on him, just in case he had a blockage in his system (they sometimes can ingest substrate).

The next day I offered Mooch his favourite foods, but he wasn't interested. Thinking, at first, that it was simply a case of his not being hungry, when the same thing happened the next day, I grew concerned. He had never refused food before.

On Tuesday I gave Mooch a warm bath, not sure whether I was worrying over nothing, though I knew that something was not right. The warm bath was supposed to stimulate his body to defecate, which would release anything that may have been lodged inside, and hopefully prompt him to eat. He was his usual lively self in the bath (something he had regularly), and we played together. He especially seemed to enjoy treading water under the shower: I suppose it may have seemed like rain or a waterfall.

I put him to bed as normal, and told him that on Wednesday I would take him to see James, our vet. I cuddled him – tighter and longer than usual for some reason – and told him that I loved him, as I always did. I stroked him a lot and, as I closed the door, said I would see him in the morning.

I came downstairs the following morning to find that he had passed away in the night. My howl of grief woke the entire family, who came running to find out what was wrong. I sat with Mooch on my lap, holding him, holding his hand and stroking it, telling him how much I loved him. I knew without doubt that I would never have another relationship with an animal like that I had had with Mooch, who had been gifted to me to demonstrate what was possible between a human and an animal of another species.

I was beyond devastated at Mooch's death, and wanted to know why? What had I done wrong?

I spoke to a friend and arranged for a university professor at a veterinary college to perform a necropsy (autopsy) on Mooch to determine the cause of death. This was particularly hard, as it meant I could not keep Mooch's body, and the photographs of the results were very hard to see. Mooch's death was caused by the way he had been cared for – the poor diet and lack of UV light – whilst with his previous owner. He had died of fatty liver disease.

In the days that followed his passing I found it difficult to sleep. One cold winter night that shone with stars I was outside at about 3am, smoking (I'm glad to say I have stopped now). Looking up at the stars, I decided to name one after Mooch, and chose the constellation of Orion, because Mooch was such a big personality and a special animal. At that moment, I felt Mooch brush against me, just the slightest breeze, on an otherwise still, cold, clear winter's night, kissing my cheek on the side of my face that I always held him against. This gave me such comfort, to know he was with me then, and is with me still, and it's the same with all animals. They are the breeze caressing our skin, the rain that falls around us, the rustle of the leaves, and the song of the birds.

Now, whenever I want, I can look up at the sky to see Mooch, and say hello to him. We talk a lot; I speak to him most nights, and he visits me often. Sometimes he is a shooting star; other times he is a breeze, or a smell that greets me when I am doing some mundane task in the house. I know it is him, letting me know he is always there, watching and guiding me, a part of me forever.

A poem that I wrote when Mooch passed away on January 12, 2012 can be found on page 81. I always feel very emotional when I read it.

5
Wasabi – The African Pygmy Hedgehog

Wasabi, also known as 'Nuclear Horseradish,' is a plant with a thick, green root that is part of the horseradish family, commonly used as a condiment in Japanese dishes; most notably sushi. It is well known for its hot and spicy flavour: proper wasabi is said to be so strong that just twelve molecules on the tongue will cause your head to explode! Much of the wasabi used in the west comes from America, and is much milder.

Having explained what wasabi is, don't you think that it's a great name for a Hedgehog? Sadly, I cannot take credit for the name: that has to go to the couple I re-homed him from – Alan Audrain and Laurent Langlais – who are now firm friends. The Hedgehog is a hot and spicy critter – hard to handle! This is the image that they want to give for protection, but it could not be further from the truth.

Hedgehogs are, by their very nature, shy animals. They are nocturnal, and therefore do not often encounter people. Because of this, when they do come across people they tend to roll into a ball, and flex their muscles, thereby becoming rather unapproachable! Flexing their muscles causes the Hedgehog's spines to become rigid, preventing them from being unrolled. The spines are strong; so strong, in fact, that one spine can support the animal's entire weight.

As already stated, I have rescued four Hedgehogs, three of whom were children's pets. Wasabi was not one of these, however, as he actually had a very loving home with Alan and Laurent, two lovely people who treated their Hedgehog like royalty, part of the reason for which was that theirs was not Wasabi's first home.

Alan and Laurent were living in Central London, in a one-bedroom apartment. Despite a lack of space, the pair felt that they had plenty of love to give a companion animal. They wanted something a little different and original, and, after initially considering a miniature pig, they decided upon a 'hog,' and set about finding one. Laurent was self-employed and worked at home, so therefore had time to dedicate to a new addition.

Unleashing the healing power of animals

Alan located a rescue Hedgehog called Brownie, who was a year old, and went to meet Brownie one evening. Alan got the impression that Brownie was 'grumpy and antisocial' – hogs huff and puff, and sound very much like an angry steam train! He was told by the current owner that the Hedgehog had been 'abused' by his first owner, and, although shy at first, soon became playful. Given this reassurance, Alan and Laurent decided to offer Brownie a home.

On getting their new pet home, however, the couple soon discovered that Brownie actually was grumpy 24/7, and was not in any way the lovely bundle of joy they had hoped for. Brownie's attitude was, in the main, because he had not received the care and attention he needed from his previous owners. If an animal does not meet the expectations of his or her owners, sadly, it is often the case that they are moved on and re-homed. This is a great shame because, with a little time and patience, any animal can become a wonderful companion, giving 100% to a relationship in terms of fun and love.

Alan and Laurent quickly discovered that Hedgehogs can be a real

Wasabi – The African Pygmy Hedgehog

pain (quite literally), and a handful! Every attempt to hold Brownie and show him love was met by a ball of firm spikes and very sore hands. In addition, they found that the animal was true to his nocturnal nature, and only really made an appearance at night. They decided to rename their ball of spikes after the sharpest, spiciest condiment in the world – Wasabi! – which really suited the Hedgehog, and is a brilliant name for this critter.

Alan and Laurent invested a lot of time and money in Wasabi, buying him a large playpen to encircle his cage, and provide him with his own territory, plus a large wheel to exercise in, and always ensured that he had the best food, even taking to breeding their own bugs and worms to ensure Wasabi's food was of the best quality. This Hedgehog had a five star, almost celebrity, lifestyle; he wanted for nothing.

Along the way the couple made many discoveries about Hedgehogs, some of them very surprising. For example, it transpired that Wasabi really liked his wheel; so much so that he ran on it all night long! Hogs will actually travel between five and seven miles a night looking for food, and snuffling in the hedgerows. They also discovered the messy and rather smelly nature of Hedgehogs, who are rather difficult to litter train (in fact, I have never met a litter-trained Hedgehog), and would awake each morning to Hedgehog poo all over their linoleum floor (which, they found, is corrosive, as well as very malodorous!). A tarpaulin was purchased to cover the floor in Wasabi's playpen, which could be easily removed and cleaned whilst he slept during the day. His exercise wheel also required daily cleaning, as Wasabi would poo as he ran, creating even more mess.

Bleach had to be used to clean the items to get them properly clean. Now, Hedgehogs react to strange smells in a strange way. Because the odours are suspicious, they do something called 'anointing' to mask their own scent, and this involves the production of thick and sticky saliva, with which they cover their spines, even those right at the back. It was Archilocus, a Greek poet (c660 BC) who, referring to this practice, said: "The fox has many tricks, but the Hedgehog has only one, and that is the best of all." When our wild Hedgehogs feel threatened, they will chew on the leaves of toxic plants (such as deadly nightshade), mixing the plant sap with their special saliva, and then anoint themselves with this, so that a predator will be spiked in the mouth or elsewhere, and end up feeling very ill because of the toxic saliva.

Alan and Laurent desperately wanted Wasabi to become their companion animal in the true sense of the word, spending time with him as a member of their family unit. After two years of trying, however, they were forced to move away from the country, and could not take Wasabi with them. This saddened them greatly, but they were determined that Wasabi would go to a home that would care for him in a way that their much-loved hog deserved. Which is where I entered the picture.

Alan and Laurent had been following my company, Critterish Allsorts, and our work on Facebook for a good while. When the time came to find a new home for Wasabi, the couple contacted me and asked if I would take him. I already had two Hedgehogs, and was happy to take a third, even though this new one was still grumpy and anti-social, refusing to uncurl and be petted.

My other Hedgehogs were regularly employed in my work: at that time this was birthday parties and fayres and fetes, as well as educational and pet therapy work. Once Hedgehogs get to know a person they tend to become more social. The Hedgehog works a lot on scent, spending hours snuffling around in hedgerows sniffing out slugs, snails, beetles, fallen fruits, and other foodstuffs. It is imperative, therefore, that when handling a Hedgehog you do not wear gloves (except with wild hogs who should always be handled wearing gloves or wrapped in a towel to avoid leaving your scent on them), because they cannot smell who is handling them. They will recognise your voice, but, having poor eyesight, will not recognise your face. In order to 'desensitise' Wasabi to being approached and touched by people, I first had to get him to feel comfortable with me. To do this I handled him with bare hands from the moment I had him, always making sure that his spines were free from faeces first.

Next, I began to talk to him, reassuringly and in a gentle and quiet voice. Hedgehogs are very sensitive to sound, and can hear at much lower volume levels than us – a normal speaking voice, can sound exceptionally loud and frightening to a Hedgehog, causing him to tightly curl into a ball. In order to habituate Wasabi to my voice, and learn to trust the sound of it, I talked to him a lot, sitting on the sofa with him cupped in my hands, gently coaxing him to relax by moving the tops of my thumbs over the spikes on his shoulders, hoping that he would find this soothing and reassuring.

I continued with this for months before getting any reaction, but, eventually, Wasabi began to uncurl. At first his nose would poke out to sniff the air, making the huffing noise that hogs are noted for, and sniffing my finger or palm to check my scent. Once he was happy he knew whose hands he was in, I would first feel his spines relax, and then his body – but only the sides, which I stroked as I talked to him, his nose right in front of my face.

The last part of Wasabi to uncurl was the flap of skin that hogs have just above their eyes (visualise a pair of particularly spiky eyebrows above a forehead that folds in on itself, and that about describes this). Although they cannot see particularly well, they are very protective of their eyes, and, once uncovered, any strange sound or movement results in the forehead collapsing and the eyebrows being pulled down over the eyes so that just the nose is evident. This was the stage I was at with Wasabi.

Once Wasabi realised that he was safe with me, sudden movement and sound ceased to worry him. He seemed to recognise my scent, voice and breath. Holding him slightly aloft, I would look up at him, and talk in a very calm and gentle voice, reassuring him that everything was okay.

Wasabi – The African Pygmy Hedgehog

Within seconds he would begin to uncurl, and he would allow me to stroke his nose, his entire body relaxed and at ease. He had got used to various noises, knowing they would not harm him, which meant that he was happy to come out and explore his surroundings, whatever time of day it was.

Wasabi then began to work alongside me, and did so for just over two years, before he died in his sleep at a little over five years old: a good age for a Hedgehog. He did not suffer any health problems, and was an extremely happy and active Hedgehog.

During the time that Wasabi and I were together, Alan and Laurent continued to visit when they could, and followed his progress on social media. They were astounded at how well and how quickly he became a therapy animal, and began to help people, but very proud of their former pet's achievements; happy that they had made the right decision in asking me to take him on.

In therapy, Wasabi was really popular, albeit he was an unusual animal to use in therapy. Having Wasabi as a therapy animal allowed many patients who loved to watch Hedgehogs enjoy a really personal, close experience, that was also very tactile. Wasabi caused giggles and laughter wherever he went, because of his spikes: people would nervously touch him, and if he then decided to stiffen his spines, this would surprise them, causing laughter all round. A delightful memory of a delightful critter.

Part of the reason why therapy animals are so beneficial is that those receiving the therapy identify with them, be this as a result of childhood experiences of feeding wild Hedgehogs, watching nature programmes on television, or from having read the wonderful Beatrix Potter books. It could even be as a result of playing a video game, such as Sonic The Hedgehog! All of these exposures and memories can trigger an affinity with an animal and explain why Wasabi was so popular in sessions. Of course, older patients suffering dementia and Alzheimer's disease probably remember experiencing these things with their children, and certainly Hedgehogs were much more abundant in gardens, for instance. When I was a boy, growing up in the 1970s, you would see Hedgehogs every night.

Meeting a Hedgehog is a significantly positive encounter for all age groups and abilities, energising the mind and providing something different to talk or write about, or even be creative about. For example, one of the images in this book shows a picture of Wasabi amongst some of the other animals who visited that residence, and was drawn for me by a dementia patient. Along with this and other pieces of art, I have poems written by patients in psychiatric hospitals, as well as models of some of my animals that have been made for me. This is the evidence – along with the obvious improvement in individuals – that lets me know that animal assisted therapy helps those with mental health issues overcome their problems, and become better able to cope with life.

6
Frostie – The Corn Snake

Frostie is a Snow Corn, and the question I am most often asked, when talking about him, is "What *is* a 'snow corn'?"

The Snow Corn is a pure albino snake, bred in captivity purely for the pet trade: a beautiful, very striking type of Corn Snake. Mainly white in colour, with pinks and yellows in the markings, they have bright pink eyes and a darker pink tongue. An albino animal has no colour pigment in the skin or eyes. Many different variations of the Snow Corn are available within the pet trade.

Corn Snakes are probably the most popular pet snake with those new to the hobby, as well as one of the most widely available. With reptiles becoming more popular as pets, the demand is there for a choice in terms of colour and pattern, which has resulted in breeders – both commercial and private – creating 'morphs': snakes selectively bred to look a certain way, to increase appeal. At the last count there were around 630 different morphs or variations of Corn Snake: that's 630 different colours/patterns! This does not mean to say that pet shops carry them all, or that you can go to a pet shop and thumb through a catalogue to choose a snake, but it does mean that a lot of snakes exist who are waiting for homes of their own.

A female snake will normally breed once a year, and lay a clutch of 15-20 eggs. After factoring in the mortality rate, this may equate to ten to 15 young. If all 630 morphs breed annually, then 6000-10,000 baby snakes are born every year, at least!

Little wonder, then, that Corn Snakes are one of the most 'unwanted' snakes. I have rescued several, and receive many requests (at least one a month) to re-home others. If I rescued every Corn Snake I was asked to, I would have well over a hundred by now!

Given the number of different morphs in existence, it's no surprise, either, that each snake I have rescued is a different colour.

Snakes become unwanted for various reasons –

- Owners do not research beforehand what's involved in keeping these animals, and subsequently find they cannot cope. They may not realise, for instance, that a diet of dead mice is required

- People buy snakes as babies (when they are small), and do not appreciate how big they can grow. Reaching an unacceptable length is one reason they become unwanted

- Conversely, some owners are impatient for their baby snake to grow to full size, and will re-home the animal because 'He isn't growing quickly enough'!

- An inability to handle snakes properly can result in the snake biting, whereupon he or she is deemed 'vicious' and moved on

- No thought is given to who will care for the animal in an owner's absence ... which is how Frostie came to join my menagerie

All of the above obstacles and problems can be overcome by research and education, via the internet and books, allowing a potential owner to make an educated decision about acquiring. When I purchased my first Skunk, for example, I carried out two years of research: not just on Skunks as an animal (ie diet, environment, etc), but also on what life with a Skunk would be like. I spoke with existing owners, breeders, zoo keepers; I went and met Skunks in domestic settings. In this way I was able to envisage what it might be like to have a Skunk as part of the family, and make my decision armed with all of the facts.

As already noted, Frostie became part of my family due to an inconsiderate owner. One summer's afternoon my phone rang.

"Hello," said a rather breathless male voice, "Is this the animal man?"

"Yes," I replied (nobody uses my name, even though it is written on my business card, website and shirt: you get used to it!). "What can I do for you?"

"I've got this white snake. I just found it in the field at the back of my house. Can you come and get it, please?"

This was a little unusual: a white snake, in a field, in rural Staffordshire. My first thought was that it might be a very rare Albino Grass Snake or Adder.

I asked the caller to describe the reptile. The snake had "very shiny skin," apparently, which told me that it was neither of these native snakes. Intrigued, I took the man's address and went to investigate further.

Arriving at the address I'd been given I was presented with a snake in a box – a very frightened and unhappy snake, who was frantically searching for a way out of the plastic box. The snake was indeed white, about as thick as my index finger, and around two feet long. It was most definitely an albino, and I identified it as a Corn Snake – a young one.

Talking with the man, it transpired that the snake belonged to a neighbour who had just gone on holiday to Italy. Apparently, the snake's owner had been asking around the neighbourhood for someone to take care of the snake whilst he was away, but without success. Subsequently, he simply released the snake into the wild to fend for himself.

The snake stuck out like a sore thumb in the grass. I have to be particularly careful when I have Frostie in the garden in the summer, as birds of prey regularly circle above our house, and it would be only a matter of seconds before he was spotted by the birds. Of course, I never take him outside if I know there are birds in the area.

Sadly, Corn Snakes are often abandoned in the wild to fend for themselves, and also sometimes escape from unsecured enclosures. Corn Snakes, native to North America, can survive in the wild when it's not cold by feeding on small rodents, but it is debatable whether they could survive a harsh British winter, for example. And even if they did, and were to breed, say, there's no guarantee that ambient temperatures would be conducive to egg incubation.

It's not beyond the realms of possibility, though, that a small population could become established in the wild. Tales exist of snakes going missing, only to turn up the following year, or even as long as 12 years later! All animals are incredibly adaptable.

And so Frostie came to live with us and our other animals. Although our relationship was a little fraught to begin with – Frostie had been understandably frightened by his experience, and had obviously not been handled regularly, in addition – he soon became quite docile with regular handling and attention, and quickly of the right temperament to become a part of the therapy team.

Frostie's first engagement was a group session with some disabled children one Christmastime, and he turned out to be a rather appropriately named critter: substitute 'Snow Corn' for 'Snowman' in the song 'Frostie The Snowman' and you'll understand why! Due to his name and his colour, the children automatically associated Frostie with Christmas, and were very happy to meet him. He was a resounding success and the children benefited from some Frostie therapy. He has been a regular ever since.

Animal assisted therapy using snakes is not particularly common, but I began doing this in 2011. Due to the stigma attached to them – and the irrational fear that many have of snakes – they're not immediately the most popular of my therapy animals. Quite often, though, it will be the staff, rather than patients, who will turn and walk out of a room when confronted by a snake, and one of the reasons for this is cultural in nature. Many of the staff working within psychiatric hospitals are of African descent. Africa is a continent that possesses a rich and diverse wildlife, amongst which are some of the world's most deadly snakes. When they are young, African children are taught a very healthy fear of and respect for all snakes – because if an encounter with one goes wrong, it's possible to end up dead. As a result, African adults are naturally fearful of snakes.

I manage this attitude by helping members of staff face and overcome their fear or phobia, and generally find that they embrace the beauty and nature of snakes once this happens. The snakes' popularity then increases as a result, and Frostie is regularly requested for therapy sessions.

The effect that a snake has on those in therapy is three-dimensional, and particularly effective for people with self-esteem issues, and even those suffering depression, to some extent.

The first dimension is how the snake feels to the individual, not just through touch, but more importantly their movement. Snakes move by muscular contraction – almost like a Mexican wave flowing along their body – which imparts a squeeze/release sensation to those they are lying on. When handling snakes in therapy, I teach people to 'be like a tree' – *they* don't hold a snake, a snake holds *them* – because, to all intents and purposes, they *are* tree-like to a snake: the body is the trunk and the arms are limbs. Snakes are happy to relax on and around an arm, and equally happy to explore an entire body!

Once the snake is established and comfortable with the patient, the rest of the therapy can begin. Whilst the squeeze/release sensation can relax a person, much like a gentle massage would, if the snake stops moving, relaxes, and remains still on a patient, then a feeling of 'belonging' and love results: "He likes me" is often heard at this stage, and this is, in some ways, true. To feel safe and accepted by an animal who is often feared and vilified is a very powerful emotion.

Secondly, it's suggested that the patient stroke the snake, just as with any other animal, such as a dog or a cat. Doing so feels just as nice, and it releases the same feel good endorphins, including serotonin and oxytocin. In addition, another chemical is released within the brain when patients take therapy with a snake – dopamine – which is triggered by the 'fight or flight' response that is instinctive in all animals when we are fearful or excited. It's how we might feel when riding a roller coaster: thrilled and animated.

The third and final dimension involves boosting confidence and self-esteem.

Those with low self-esteem within psychiatric institutions, seem to find themselves socially isolated, to a degree, and low down within the patient hierarchy. Holding a snake in a room full of people who cannot believe how brave they are being boosts their standing, as those at a higher hierarchical level develop an immediate respect for their fellow patient, who is willing to do something that they are not. Doctors, occupational therapists and other staff are also astounded by their charge's bravery in the face of such a challenge. All of this new-found respect and admiration is voiced by those present – patients and medical professionals alike – elevating the low-esteem patient's standing. Praise, respect and a whole new positivity comes their way because they interacted with a snake, and they leave a session feeling accomplished, confident, positive, and happy. And of course, the more often they experience this, the greater these feelings of worthiness become, until the patient's self-esteem is permanently boosted; not just in *their* minds, but also in those of their peers. It can be a real life changer.

There are also particular benefits for those with psychosis, as therapy with a snake leaves them feeling thrilled, excited and calm, all at the same time, which really helps with management of their condition.

Frostie also promotes feelings of empathy from those he meets. Many of the adults and children with issues I deal with seem to really relate to his story of being abandoned by his human 'parents' (we humanise our pets all of the time, referring to ourselves as 'mommy' or 'daddy,' and their relationship to our children as their 'sister' or 'brother,' etc), and left to fend for himself. Along with this, snakes carry a certain stigma, just as those with mental health issues can, which, again, patients identify with. In some cases, getting past the stigma attached to snakes is symbolic or representative of overcoming the stigma surrounding their mental health issues: if they can do it, then so can others. So I guess it gives them hope for the future.

Frostie is a special snake who has helped many people in many ways to improve their lives. Hopefully, he will lead the way for more snakes to succeed in animal assisted therapy. Although the larger breeds of snake would be too cumbersome for this kind of therapy, Corn Snakes, Rat Snakes and the beautiful Rainbow Boas, with their good temperament, are just perfect. I also use Connie, my Common Boa, who is very popular due to her gentle and friendly demeanour.

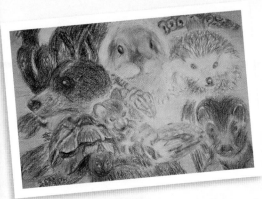

This delightful picture was drawn by a care home resident, with severe dementia. He had received several visits from the animals, and had chosen to draw this and present it to me. It was his way of thanking us for our visits, our companionship, and our help.

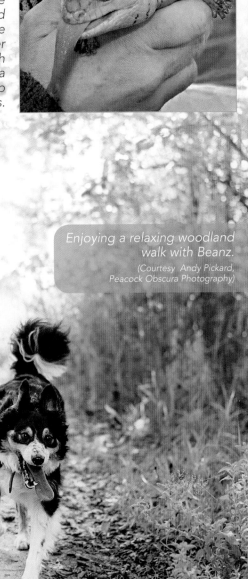

Shiver showing us how she got her name! You will also notice that the tongue has a blunt fork at the end, and the main use of this is as a defence mechanism. Fanned wide across her mouth, the colour and contrast (with the rest of the mouth), coupled with a sudden fairly loud hiss, is shocking to most predators.

Enjoying a relaxing woodland walk with Beanz.
(Courtesy Andy Pickard, Peacock Obscura Photography)

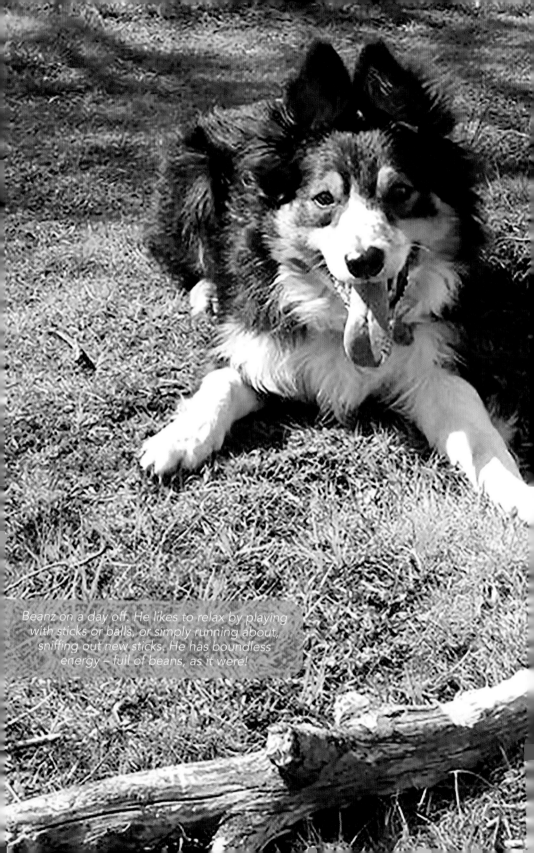

Beanz on a day off. He likes to relax by playing with sticks or balls, or simply running about, sniffing out new sticks. He has boundless energy – full of beans, as it were!

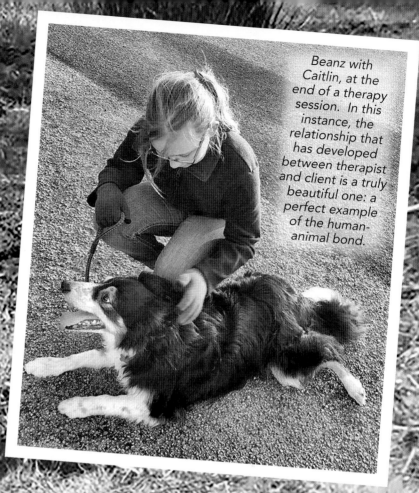

Beanz with Caitlin, at the end of a therapy session. In this instance, the relationship that has developed between therapist and client is a truly beautiful one: a perfect example of the human-animal bond.

Tinkerbell 'fixing things' in her own inimitable way ...

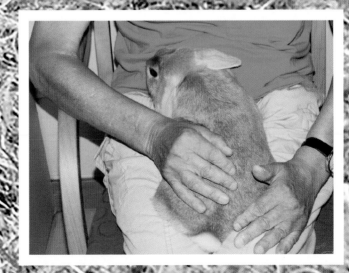

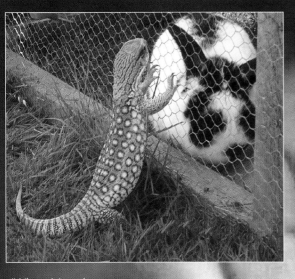

'When Mooch met Joseph.' Mooch was always curious – he was just a baby when this was taken.

A Millipede: many legs make light work of hypersensitive skin: insects helping people to welcome physical contact.

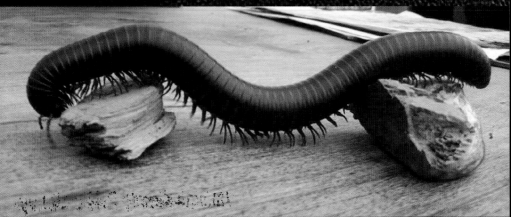

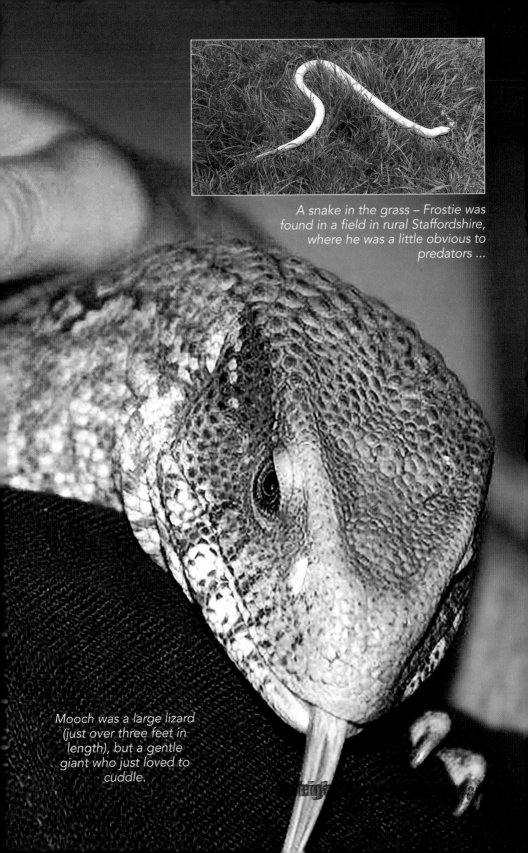

A snake in the grass – Frostie was found in a field in rural Staffordshire, where he was a little obvious to predators ...

Mooch was a large lizard (just over three feet in length), but a gentle giant who just loved to cuddle.

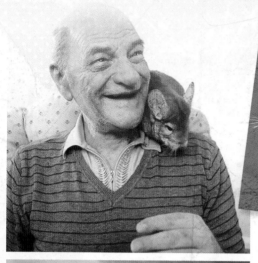

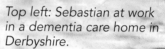

Top left: Sebastian at work in a dementia care home in Derbyshire.
(Courtesy Sophie Wedgewood, sophiewedgewood.com)

Top right: Posing for professional photographs did not faze Sebastian at all!
(Courtesy Andy Pickard, Peacock Obscura Photography)

Left: Sebastian with me at a weekend Scout and Guide camp, where we put the attendees through a sensory educational workshop. I asked the questions and Sebastian provided the exciting and fun sensory stimulus!
(Courtesy Andy Pickard, Peacock Obscura Photography)

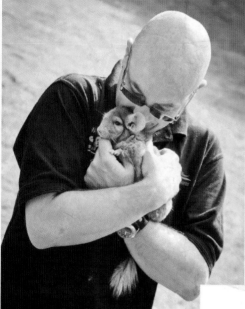

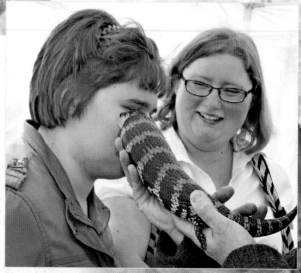

Shiver giving a young blind adult a sensory experience by 'kissing' her on the cheek. In addition the girl also stroked and held Shiver.

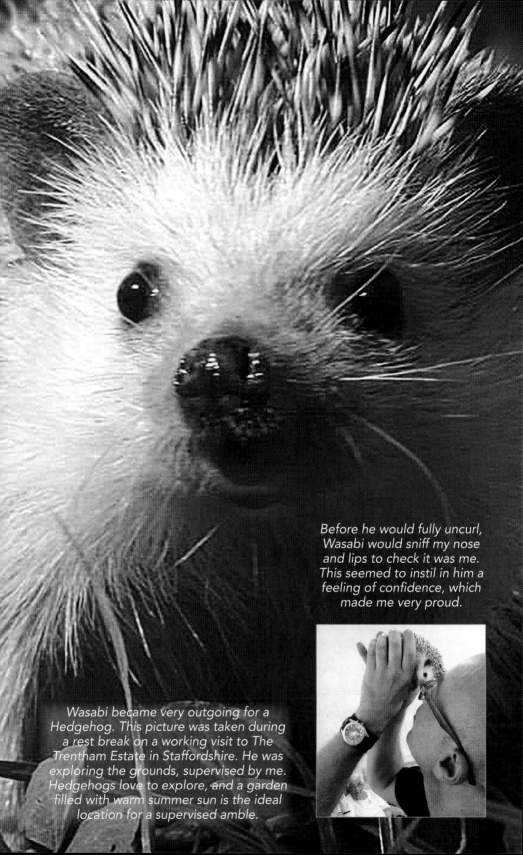

Before he would fully uncurl,
Wasabi would sniff my nose
and lips to check it was me.
This seemed to instil in him a
feeling of confidence, which
made me very proud.

Wasabi became very outgoing for a
Hedgehog. This picture was taken during
a rest break on a working visit to The
Trentham Estate in Staffordshire. He was
exploring the grounds, supervised by me.
Hedgehogs love to explore, and a garden
filled with warm summer sun is the ideal
location for a supervised amble.

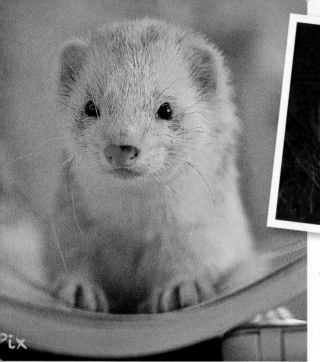

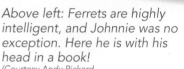

Above left: Ferrets are highly intelligent, and Johnnie was no exception. Here he is with his head in a book!
(Courtesy Andy Pickard,
Peacock Obscura Photohgraphy)

Above: Let sleeping Ferrets lie: Ferrets can sleep for up to 20 hours a day – the Ferret equivalent of teenagers!

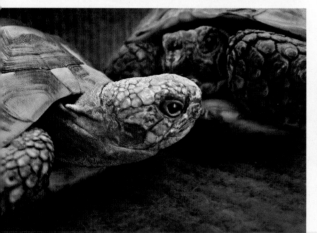

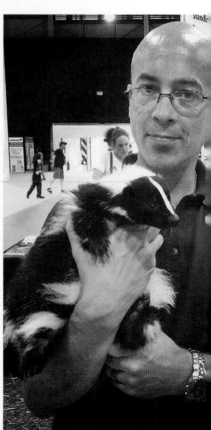

Tortoises in conversation – we have two Tortoises at Critterish Allsorts: George, the Hermann's, and Moshi, who is a Horsefield. Here they are seen in rare conversation with each other: generally, George is chasing Moshi (who is twice his size) away from his 'patch.' Wonder what they talk about ...?

Stoosh and I at a show, where the public got to learn all about Skunks and their value as therapy animals. Stoosh has the ability to firstly make most people sit up and take notice ... and then melt in delight!

7
George – The Hermann's Tortoise

George is a Hermann's Tortoise. There are several varieties of Hermann's Tortoise, all of which can be found in Europe, mainly around the eastern Mediterranean coast, and especially in Italy, Greece, and Turkey. They are protected by CITES (the Convention on International Trade in Endangered Species [of Flora & Fauna]), an agreement between international governments to ensure that international trade in specimens of animals and plants does not endanger their survival in the wild. This means that, in order to live with a CITES-protected animal, a licence and a microchip are required. The licence shows the bloodline of your animal, and proves that they are descended from captive-bred animals, and not taken from the wild. The microchip allows the animal to be traced to you, should they go missing.

George came to us from Europe – Germany, to be exact. It was a weekday when the phone rang. The well-spoken young lady on the other end had a bit of a dilemma. As a teenager, she lived in Germany with her parents (her father was in the armed forces and stationed there). During her childhood, they had moved all over Europe, and she had fallen in love with the wild Tortoises they had seen. As she grew up, she asked her father if they could have a Tortoise as a pet. Eventually, her father gave in to her requests (as they invariably do), and bought her a Tortoise as a pet – a Hermann's Tortoise, that she named George.

A few years later, the family returned to the UK and was stationed in Staffordshire. Fast forward to the present day and George's owner had a

LEGAL MATTERS
If purchasing a Tortoise from a retailer as a pet, be sure about the species of the animal you are buying, and if this is a licensed variety, be sure to receive your A10 licence at the same time. If the animal is gifted to you, however, there is no legal requirement to have a licence.

The law is strange, sometimes!

problem: her boyfriend had relocated to Australia, and she wanted to be with him. Tortoises don't travel so well, however, which meant that poor George could not tag along with her (it also transpired that Australia was not keen on allowing migrant Tortoises citizenship).

She told me that she had followed my company for a couple of years, and recognised the love we had for our animals. She wondered if we would accept George into our family, because she felt that he would have the perfect home with us.

When somebody shows that kind of trust in you, it's extremely heart-warming, as you realise that this is the perceived public image of you and your company. Of course, I said yes to taking George on one condition: that we would foster George until such time as the young lady had decided whether or not to stay in Australia. If things did not work out and she returned to the UK, then she and George could be reunited. I've not heard whether or not the move proved successful, but we still have George! I do know, however, that she keeps an eye on George's progress from time-to-time, and monitors his work.

According to his licence, George was born in August 2008, and arrived here with us around four years ago (circa 2012), happily growing with us and continuing to do so. About 12 months after he arrived, he was big enough to receive his microchip (Tortoises must be at least 60mm in diameter to be microchipped). Now, imagine if you will, a Tortoise of this size (less than 3 inches) being implanted with a microchip just like the ones used for dogs and cats! Unfortunately, it's a legal requirement with certain species. There is a liquid (the latest in forensic science), used by the police, which can be painted onto the shell of a Tortoise to link it to a specific address. The liquid is non-toxic and hard-wearing, meaning that it cannot be washed or rubbed off, and contains a unique code. As with a microchip, the code is registered to an address, ensuring that the animal is traceable to its owner. It costs about the same as microchipping, and is greatly preferable to the microchipping process, which is quite invasive and, I would imagine, painful, too.

Watching George being microchipped was a little traumatic for me, never mind him and his little leg (which is where the chip is implanted), and the same size needle and chip are used for a Tortoise as for a cat or a dog. Anyone who has seen their pet receive a microchip will appreciate how uncomfortable this can be. Tortoises have no flesh to speak of under their skin, which tears easily as a result: as the vet pushed the needle into George's back leg, a small tear appeared, through which I could see the leg's internal workings.

Once the microchip was implanted, the vet had to repair the tear, and what did he use? Superglue, which, according to my vet, was developed for soldiers in the Vietnam war, who would carry it in their packs, so that, if injured in the jungle, they could use this to seal a wound and get to hospital. Happily, George's ordeal seemed not to bother him at all, and it was only me who was traumatised by the process, leaving a memory I will never get out of my head!

George's first experience of the public was at a birthday party (which I soon realised is not a good environment for my animals, so stopped doing these). Whether at a birthday party or a school, whenever a Tortoise appears, it is usually greeted by cries of 'Turtle!' and I quickly explain that George is a Tortoise, NOT a turtle! There is a marked difference, although many people do not know what that difference is, so I go on to explain this, too. (It's good to hear the children later explain to their mystified parents the difference between a turtle and Tortoise.) Thanks to Teenage Mutant Ninja Turtles, any creature with a shell is a turtle, especially as far as children are concerned. In American-English, the term 'turtle' is used to describe the entire order of Testudines – an order of reptiles which comprises turtles, terrapins, and Tortoises – (or Chelonii: a suborder of Testudinata, comprising all the land and fresh-water forms), whereas in Britain, 'turtle' is used to describe those animals which dwell in the water, whilst those that dwell on land are called 'Tortoises.'

George has always been a confident Tortoise, and has never once withdrawn into his shell when in public. His size also wins hearts, as, being just 8 years old, he is quite small and cute-looking. Having said that, he has grown quite a lot since he arrived at Critterish Cottage just a few years ago, as he can certainly eat! Tortoises can eat as much food at each meal as could be fitted into their upturned shell, and George is no exception as he clears his plate in a flash – and they say Tortoises are slow!

Tortoises can move, too, especially where food is involved. They have a keen sense of smell, and George will pick out his favourite foods – such as cucumber and apple – first. Opinion is divided about how well Tortoises can hear, but, when called, George readily responds. Tortoises have a fully developed inner ear, but no outer ear, and it is known that they can discern a lower frequency range than can we, which overlaps with our range, meaning that we can hear some of the same sounds. There is no doubt, though, that George knows his name – especially when food is in the offing.

George is very loyal, too, and I have read a few accounts from people who share their lives with Tortoises who have found the same. When he is out and about in the house or the garden and I am in the same area, George will come and sit on my foot whilst I work. It is a very endearing trait, and adds to his already amazing character, although it can also be a little inconvenient ...

A question I am often asked is whether Tortoises can feel when things are done to their shell, or it is touched (the carapace is the upper shell and the plastron is the lower (underneath) shell). George had been well cared for before he came to me, but I have seen some rescue cases whose shells have been in really bad condition, and sometimes as a result of damage from foxes or dogs. The shell *is* sensitive, and is made of the same material as are our hair and nails: beneath the top layer of shell are nerve endings, just like we have beneath our nails, so a Tortoise can feel every scratch, stroke or rub of their shell.

True to form, George demonstrates his appreciation of attention in his own special way. Tickle him on the plate (or scute) above his head and he will push against your finger, much as a cat will do when their head is stroked. His favourite, though, is to be tickled in a circular motion at the rear of his shell. He wiggles his rear end from side-to-side in enjoyment, pushing down on his foot and up with his leg at the same time. It's hilarious to watch – this Tortoise has character by the bucket-load!

Going on what I have told you so far about this happy character, you can appreciate that he is quite a popular member of the therapy team, and I always take him with me when visiting care homes, for one reason in particular. Most of the residents in care homes are aged 70 and above. In the 1960s and '70s, Tortoises were very popular pets in the UK, and almost every family had one. *Blue Peter* – a British institution in terms of children's television shows – had a pet Tortoise on the show, which further increased the animal's popularity. Tortoises were freely available in every high street pet shop for very little cost, making them easy to find and purchase. Many older people therefore have very fond memories of Tortoises because of the situation back then, and seeing George revives happy reminiscences.

As we work with dementia and Alzheimer's patients, this is a particularly good form of therapy that helps with memory recall, sometimes winkling out memories where once there was nothing. Residents have remembered long-forgotten memories of their children playing with the family Tortoise, or of their Tortoise escaping. Sitting with their relatives, they are once again able to share fond memories of times past. One lady in particular recalled life with her husband when they bred Tortoises. It is always such a beautiful and life-affirming experience, to see a light come on in their eyes that an animal has sparked, reviving a memory buried deep, but remembered once more.

Some of my residents in care homes will only spend time with the Tortoise, and are not at all interested in the furries. They sit with George and stroke him, talking or even singing to him, and are absolutely delighted by the experience. It makes the work we do in animal assisted therapy so rewarding: there's a real sense of having helped someone by bringing something special to their day and making a difference.

In psychiatric hospitals, George has also proved his worth, where, again, his big character makes him very popular. In one instance, he really changed a patient's attitude and approach for the better. This particular patient was verbally and physically abusive to other patients and staff, as well as generally violent and aggressive. Of course, these are not desirable traits in any instance – especially not within the confines of a ward – and can result in negative treatment of the individual by staff and

George – The Hermann's Tortoise

other patients. Consequences can include fighting, bullying, physical restraint, and even isolation. Negativity breeds negativity.

Enter George!

The first time that this patient attended a session, the result was nothing short of miraculous for those who worked with and lived with him, particularly as we had been told to expect very little, and warned about his unpredictable nature. Attending with his doctor, a psychologist, the patient felt an instant connection with George, and asked if he could sit on the grass with him. It was a warm, sunny day, and, as the patient would be supervised by his doctor, a member of staff and me, I agreed to his request – George would love being on the grass, so it would be great for him, anyway.

The patient sat on the grass and placed George in front of him. He'd not stopped smiling since setting eyes on George, but now he also began talking to the Tortoise, and not in his usual, aggressive way, either, but in that sing-song way that we sometimes use with our children and animals.

"Oh, you are a beautiful boy," he said, "Aren't you a beautiful boy? All shiny and smooth. I love you." The last three words caused the psychologist's mouth to literally drop open. The patient's entire demeanour had softened, and he was relaxed. I could see, too, that the staff were also more relaxed, compared to how rigid and on guard they had been initially. Just ten minutes into therapy, George's presence was having a positive effect on the patient, immediately calming him and the surrounding environment. Staff normally spent the entire time they were with this patient on high alert, because of his tendency to become violent or aggressive, or attempt to escape. The introduction of one small animal had reduced the usual tension to virtually zero. Amazing.

That first day the patient spent a total of two hours with George. Ensuing visits and sessions – I visited him once a fortnight – were shorter, but because of their frequency the positive effects were maintained and built upon. This was a huge change for the patient, and not just him, either, but also the staff who managed him, and also his fellow patients. Everyone had seen a softer, more approachable side to his personality, allowing the realisation that there was something positive there to work with and on, by combining this new therapy with everything else they were doing, to help the patient deal with his issues and eventually rejoin society.

Life for this patient was completely turned around by a little Hermann's Tortoise by the name of George!

8
Tinkerbell – The Rabbit

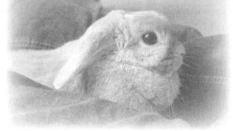

Tinkerbell (lovingly referred to by her nickname, Tink) has a story that is more sad than happy. It can also give rise to feelings of anger – so keep in mind that there is a happy ending; not just for her, but also for many who have met her, and love her.

Unlike her Disney namesake, Tink is not at all feisty, stubborn or hot-tempered: in fact, she is quite the opposite. In common with her namesake, however, she is beautiful, fair-furred, and pure of heart. She also has a little white pom-pom, though not on her shoes: hers is her tail – she has similar colouration to a wild Rabbit, with a white flash when she lifts her tail, which, in wild Rabbits, acts as a warning to others. Like Tinkerbell, she also has a love of 'lost things' (although in a different way!). As Disney Tinkerbell says: "I'm a Tinker. It's who I am, and Tinkers fix things." And, boy, does our Tinker fix things!

All of the animals featured in this book are rescues, and Tink is no exception. Her story begins when Jean saw some very cute bunnies – Dwarf Lops – for sale on a social media page, and contacted the seller to arrange a visit so that she could choose one.

Jean and I went to the seller's house, and she chose her baby Rabbit. The seller (a woman in her sixties who had lost her husband, but discovered a passion for breeding Rabbits) appeared to have a lot of Rabbits, contained in two sheds in her back garden. Unfortunately, in common with many hobbyist breeders, the woman did not have the necessary knowledge or experience to be breeding Rabbits on such a large scale, although she was quite proud of her breeding pedigree and who she supplied.

Over time, Jean got to know the breeder quite well via social media, and the woman took Jean into her confidence.

One day, she privately messaged Jean to tell her that she had a litter of Rabbits who were 'not in the best shape,' and had 'deformities.' If Jean would like one, it could be at a much lower price. Apparently,

Tinkerbell – The Rabbit

the deformities were misshapen, broken or dislocated limbs, which had occurred during birth. Jean went to take a look at the litter and returned distraught by what she had seen: baby Rabbits with horrendously-shaped limbs who could hardly walk. Most of the babies died as the breeder was not prepared to pay for veterinary treatment, but one did survive and we called him Piglet.

Piglet, we later discovered, was Tink's son, and he had problems with his front legs, which appeared to have been broken/dislocated at the knee/elbow at birth, and then fused together over the following weeks. It seems that Piglet got around by using his elbows as feet, and had adapted quite well. Our vet assured us that, although his situation was obviously not ideal, Piglet was not in any pain and was not suffering. We were also told that he could expect a shortened lifespan, but we decided to give him the best life possible in whatever time he had.

Jean certainly loved her Rabbits, there's no question about that! She doted on them, as she doted on her children, and Piglet could not have wished for a better human companion. He got special treatment, too, to ensure that his life was as enjoyable and fulfilled as it could be, enjoying playtimes with her and the children, and spending many hours playing with balls in the garden and being fed dandelions. He also came out as a therapy animal on occasion, especially when I was working with physically disabled children. As mentioned in previous chapters, children especially identified with his disabilities, and the ways in which he had adapted to live a full life.

Sadly, Piglet never really grew properly, and passed away at the age of three.

During the first couple of months of Piglet's time with us, Jean was again contacted by the breeder, who explained that she could no longer breed from Piglet's mother, as all of the kits she produced had 'disabilities.' The breeder offered us Piglet's mother, as she was no longer contributing to her business, which is how Tinkerbell became part of our family.

We discovered when we collected Tinkerbell that she was just 8 months old, by which time, she had apparently given birth to three litters, meaning that she began breeding at around three or four months of age. Although female Rabbits become sexually mature at the age of three months or thereabouts, they should not be bred until at least six months of age, to ensure that they are properly developed and big enough to cope with carrying a litter. A smaller-framed Rabbit, as Tinkerbell is, should be allowed a few extra months to ensure sufficient growth and strength.

Tinkerbell had obviously had a very poor start to life, insofar as she had been used as a 'bunny machine,' specifically to create babies that the breeder could sell. Had she not begun to have deformed kits, this misuse may have continued for several years. And Tink is not an isolated case, as many hobbyists and backyard breeders employ similar practices, using females to produce the 'cute bunnies' seen in pet stores, many of whom turn a blind eye to how their 'stock' came about.

Naturally, we were pleased that we could make a difference to at least one of these poor animals, by offering her a lifetime of love. We reported the breeder to the authorities in the hope and expectation that her business would be closed down.

And so Tinkerbell began a new life with us, and was, from the outset, gentle and quiet, with a beautiful temperament. It was obvious that she would make a perfect therapy animal, receiving lots of love and positive attention in the process, from all sorts of people.

HOMEBUDDIES
Should an animal not prove suitable for our therapy work, he or she remains with us for life, receiving just as much love and attention from us, although not, of course, meeting other people as the therapy guys do.

Have you ever looked at a Rabbit's mouth, I wonder? As you will have read in Chapter 1, my very first pet was a Rabbit, so I have a very special place in my heart for these animals. One thing I noticed about my Rabbit, Silky, was that he always looked like he was smiling, which is why I always consider Rabbits to be happy animals. I think that Tinkerbell was happy because she had been saved from a life as a breeding doe.

My critters can be regarded as 'working' animals, of course, and I consider them to be my colleagues in this – they are the true therapy-givers, after all, although they are not trained, nor put through a course or series of tests to ensure that they are 'qualified' to be a therapy animal. During my assessment of their suitability for therapy work they are shown much love and attention, and, if they are considered cut out for therapy work, they will get to meet other people who also show them love and attention, during the course of a session. These people have their own issues and in return for the love and attention they show to the therapy animal, they are helped by their therapy animal to deal with those issues. It is a simple exchange between service user and therapy animal, which is mutually beneficial.

Sadly, over time, Tinkerbell has developed other problems because of the abuse she suffered. Twice a day I check her for impacted faeces, which are a direct result of her rear end being overstretched giving birth at too early an age. I feed her only certain foods and avoid others to minimise her discomfort and prevent her from getting in a mess.

Tinkerbell was a great therapy animal from the outset, and in the time that we have been colleagues she has made a difference to so many people. I have also seen her confidence grow, and she exhibits various traits that I never would have dreamed an animal could. She is a very popular therapy animal, who has worked with everyone from small children to elderly people with dementia, and is loved by all age ranges.

Small children are drawn to her because she is cute and fluffy – her fur is almost as soft as Sebastian's, the Chinchilla, and therefore really beautiful to stroke. She has big eyes that radiate calm and knowledge, as observed and noted on by several people – teenagers who have experienced her therapy within their CAMHS (Child and Adolescent Mental Health Services) units, and older people in psychiatric hospitals. Her placid nature does not go unnoticed, either, and is, I think, part of her appeal – she is happy to sit with anyone, quietly sharing space and time. This makes her a favourite with elderly people, and nursing home staff have commented on the calm she brings to residents, who can be quite erratic in their behaviours.

These beneficial effects are experienced by the majority of those who encounter furry therapy animals, as an animal who is naturally calm creates an air of tranquillity in whatever environment they are in, which transfers to those there, be they residents, patients, or staff. The weight of an animal on a lap is relaxing, as their warmth spreads through the limbs and into the abdominal area, making the patient feel warm inside. Add to this the effects of feel good hormones that result from the action of stroking an animal, and it's the equivalent of a nice big warm hug from a loved one.

The sense of calmness that animals bring to an environment is best demonstrated during my regular visits for group sessions at a female CAMHS ward. The patients are all under the age of 18, so you can imagine the anticipation and excitement that exists in advance of our visits, which builds to a palpable buzz when we arrive on the ward, as the girls speculate about which animals have come this time, and whether their favourite is one of them. From the moment that the girls begin to interact with the animals, however, there's almost instant calm as the buzz quickly dies down.

This composure is what we need, initially, so that we can begin to work with individuals, to try and bring about the results required for that particular patient.

I mentioned earlier that Tinkerbell had developed certain traits which are unusual for an animal to have, and one in particular has not only been noticed by me, but also psychologists and care workers, who have pointed out Tinkerbell's uncanny ability when it comes to a specific mental health problem. This has been commented on and discussed at length, but there seems to be no other identifiable trigger or cause for her behaviour, and has therefore been attributed to instinct alone.

The health issue I am talking about is depression. Tinkerbell seems to know when a person is depressed, and psychologists and care workers who have worked with us for several years comment that she always seems to know just how to behave with particular patients. "Do you think that she can sense they are depressed?" they ask, or "How does your Rabbit know which patients suffer with depression? She always acts like that around depressed patients."

To explain. When someone is experiencing depression, even though there are not always obvious signs of this, somehow, Tinkerbell knows, and will climb up onto that person's chest as far as she can, and nudge their chin with her nose, as if to say 'Chin up, everything is going to be okay,' after which she will settle on their chest to be stroked, as if she also knows how soothing and beneficial this is.

This was most beautifully demonstrated with a young patient on a CAMHS ward, who, suffering with depression, was almost mute. This patient communicated via the odd muffled grunt, or by writing on a piece of paper. This was the first time that she had attended a session, usually preferring to remain in her room.

When I arrived, she was sitting alone at a table, away from the main group, and told staff that she was not interested in the session, because she did not like animals. She did remain, however, and watched as the rest of the group interacted with the animals and displayed obvious pleasure as they did so.

45 minutes or so into the one-hour session, the lone patient asked to see George, 'the tortoise,' who she interacted with a little, and for a relatively short period of time. This was a result – a small one, granted – but sometimes this is all we get in the initial stages. When the patient lost interest in George, she asked if she could see Tinkerbell, who was taken to her and placed on the table in front of her. The patient brought her head down level with Tinkerbell, who turned and faced the young girl, moving closer to place her little nose under the patient's chin, then gently lifting it. This made the patient smile, and she scooped up Tinkerbell, enveloping her in her dressing gown, against her shoulder and chest.

Miraculously, the girl then began to speak in a whisper to the member of staff she was sitting with. Mindful that something very important was happening, I extended the session to allow the breakthrough to continue.

I have no doubt that Tinkerbell will continue to be one of our most popular therapy animals with people of all ages for a long time to come.

9
Shiver – The Blue-tongued Skink

Shiver, a Blue-tongued Skink, is a ground-foraging lizard from Australia, often found in and around suburban back gardens there. The large head and chunky body are completely out of proportion to the short, skinny legs, and the large blue tongue flicks in and out of the mouth in a snake-like way. Their strange proportions mean that they are not particularly quick, and do not run: in fact, it is surprising that their legs are capable of lifting and moving their large, cumbersome bodies at all. Their main line of defence is their striking blue tongue, which they spread across their open mouth, whilst hissing loudly. The resultant contrast of blue and pink in the mouth area, coupled with the sudden and loud hiss, can be sufficient to deter attack.

Truly a strange lizard to behold, Skinks are often confused with a fish, or a snake, which I can understand in terms of evolutionary transition. It's said that every animal on earth came from the sea. As Neil Shubin, the palaeontologist who discovered Tiktaalik, the fossil of a 375 million year old fish-like creature, from which we are claimed to be descended, said, "Embrace your inner fish." I'm not sure whether Shiver does do, but I can certainly see her inner fish, so I embrace it on her behalf – her ears are often mistaken for gills by those she meets!

Shiver was living in Sheffield when I got a call in December 2010 to say she was in need of help. I don't honestly know what gender Shiver is, actually. Blue-tongued Skinks are notoriously difficult to sex without going through a pretty invasive procedure involving steel probes, so we're quite happy to believe that she is a girl! She was named by my stepdaughter, and Shiver is a reflection of the time of year – winter – that she arrived with us.

Shiver was in a bit of a state when she arrived with us in Lichfield, and it was clear from the outset that her original human companions were a little out of their depth. A Blue-tongued Skink requires pretty specialist care, especially in terms of environment, and when it comes to shedding their skin: a process that happens about three or four times a year, in Shiver's case.

On closer inspection, it could be seen that Shiver was wearing 'gloves' on each leg: three or four layers of old skin. As her environment had not had the proper humidity, she had found the shedding process very difficult, and so failed to lose all of her old skin. Skinks are composed of large, pronounced scales, some of which remained on her back and head, and had done for a long time, posing a significant risk of skin damage.

The first thing we did was bathe Shiver. We ran some warm water in an enclosed 'rub' (a box that we use for transporting our animals, which is a standard item used for transporting lizards), placed her inside and put on the lid. There was sufficient water in the rub for her to stand comfortably without fear of drowning. The water was warm enough to produce a little condensation, but not warm enough to burn her.

With the lid on, the warm water and resulting condensation created a 'humidity chamber,' or sauna, which began to work on the lodged scales. Because respiratory tract infections pose a risk to reptiles we could not leave her in the 'sauna' for too long, and after 20 minutes, she was removed and wiped dry. Some of the scales had loosened in the sauna, and the drying-off allowed them to easily come away. Others were still stuck fast, though, including the 'gloves' of skin that she was wearing around each of her feet.

For the next stage a dampened cotton bud was used to gently ease off the more stubborn scales. It's important to pay close attention to the eyelids of a Blue-tongued Skink, because if the skin does not come away from these during the shedding process, it gradually shrinks, thereby reducing blood flow to the skin, with the result that the eyelids can be lost, which means that the animal is then unable to close their eyes or blink, creating further issues with the eyes and their eyesight. This had not happened to Shiver, thankfully.

However, the situation with her 'gloved' feet was not as good.

Around four layers of skin remained on each leg – around 12 months' worth of skin that should have been shed – which had become tighter and tighter around her toes, until the blood supply had been cut off, and the ends of her toes had been lost.

Shiver's treatment continued over the next week with a 20-minute sauna every other day, and I carried on working on removing her scales. Eventually, she was scale-free, and the layers of old skin on her legs and feet had been completely removed (a very messy and time-consuming job, I can tell you!). After this, I continued to give Shiver a weekly sauna in order to condition her skin, and provide her some much-needed humidity. When she next shed her skin, although it was not perfect, it was a much easier and less time-consuming job, the skin coming off her legs and feet particularly easily, which was great news. The regular 'sauna' had worked, and we were obviously giving her what she needed in terms of environment.

After her first shed in our care, we reduced Shiver's sauna to every other week, and then once a month, when we were happy that she was shedding in a healthy manner. Today, Shiver's skin just slides off when it needs to, and all sorts of shapes can be found in her enclosure. Those we like the most are the gloves that come off her feet: dainty, now, and no longer like gauntlets! The other great thing is that, over the years, her toes have gradually grown, and she has also managed to grow a few claws on the end of some of them!

An important lesson from Shiver's story is never to underestimate what it takes to look after an animal – any animal – properly. Research, research, research, everything you can about the particular animal, and its requirements in captivity. Go and see them in the homes of others who care for them; speak to owners on forums or face-to-face; discover and understand exactly what's involved in the care of such an animal; speak to the veterinary profession, and make sure that you have a vet within easy reach who understands how to care for the animal concerned. Having done these things, only then can you be sure that you can give that animal everything they need to be healthy and happy – something that applies to ALL animals, of course, and not just the more exotic of them. In this way, hopefully, we can reduce the number of animals who find themselves in rescue centres all over the world ...

A Blue-tongued Skink can live for anything between 20 and 30 years, so are quite a commitment in terms of time as well as care. Shiver was fully grown when she came to us, and we estimated her age – based on what we were told by her previous human companions – at between seven and eight years, which means that, as I type this today, Shiver is a middle-aged 14 years old.

In terms of temperament, Blue-tongued Skinks are generally quite mild characters. Although they will hiss when approached, they will not try to run, and are quite easy to pick up, as they do not wriggle incessantly as some lizards do, and are relatively calm once picked up. When holding these lizards, if they feel as though they are on firm ground, they will be still when held. We therefore support Shiver's feet if she is not on somebody's lap, on the floor of a room, or on the ground in a garden.

One of the most important things to remember when using animals in therapy, of course, is that their comfort and safety is the first consideration. During sessions, if either of these seem compromised in any way, the session does not go ahead, or carry on if already begun.

Shiver has always done well as a therapy animal, and has never exhibited any kind of negative behaviour: she is one of the most popular animals; requested by young and old alike. When in a session, Shiver is happy to be held and stroked, or to sit on a lap and be stroked. She sits proudly, with her head held high, and enjoys all of the attention that comes her way. She does seem to be an immensely proud lizard, and who can blame her? She is beautiful to behold, has a fine temperament, and will even give kisses. Everyone she meets is fascinated by everything about her – her tongue, her shape, her legs ... and even how she evolved, a subject which can be the start of many good-natured and lengthy conversations.

I think that she has a certain mystique about her, but she is chosen more often than not because of her quirky appearance. Some people with specific mental health issues, such as paranoia and psychosis, are particularly drawn to her, for reasons I am yet to discover, but this lizard certainly appears to have a calming effect. As mentioned previously, it's well known that stroking and petting any animal will release endorphins into the blood stream that have a soothing effect, just as stroking a soft-coated or furry animal will.

But, as with a snake, there is an element of overcoming a natural fear about being in close contact with another reptile. Shiver is not a small lizard at around 18 inches long, and bulky with it. Nevertheless, her resemblance to a snake is such that she is often mistaken for one, especially given her short, spindly legs, which are not very obvious. Her oral anatomy is different to that of a snake: her mouth and tongue work in a different way, and, in order to flick out her tongue she must first open her mouth, an action considered quite challenging by many, who fear she may bite them. But overcoming any aversion to her is very beneficial to those suffering self-esteem issues, who often finish a session on a high, with a heightened sense of self-worth for the same reasons they do when spending time with Frostie, the Corn Snake.

Different people choose different animals for different reasons for their therapy, and quite why Shiver is so popular is yet to be fully understood, but she is by far the most requested reptile amongst my critters. I think the reason for her popularity is two-fold. Firstly, Shiver is absolutely beautiful to look at, and a joy to be around, and, secondly, many patients identify with her background of being mistreated, neglected, and ultimately abandoned. Patients feel sympathetic to her story, and empathise with her, wanting to let her know that she is adored by all.

Patients often joke that they would like to have Shiver and keep her in their room. "She'll be no trouble," they joke, "She'll get lots of cuddles." "I'll look after her," is another oft-heard comment. Shiver makes a big impression on these troubled minds, teaching them love and compassion, and how to laugh again. And with laughter comes a lighter atmosphere, positive social interactions, and relaxed, happy patients.

10
Johnnie – The Ferret

Ferrets have a reputation for being vicious, calculating and cold ... oh, and smelly! Having both Skunks and Ferrets within my therapy animals, I can quite confidently say that, on the smelly scale, Ferrets win, as they are more consistently smelly. Skunks only smell if they are scared, very scared, and even then it is the liquid they eject from their glands that smells rather than the Skunk. Most of the time a Skunk smells sweet and clean, like a rabbit or a cat. This is not the case with Ferrets, however, as they have a permanent, deep musky odour which is secreted onto their skin from glands near the anus. Neutering an animal can help control this smell a little, but it will always be there. It's not a strong smell, especially, and, for me, it becomes comforting when cuddling your Ferret.

FERRET FACTS

Ferrets are obligate carnivores, and can eat only meat. They have strong jaws that lock onto prey/food when they bite, and, as they have sharp teeth, this can be quite painful. Playing with a Ferret can mean being bitten sometimes, but this comes with the territory. The trick (and it's the same with any animal) is to understand the animal and his or her motivation. To your pet, you are a member of their species, and they will therefore interact with you as such.

Ferrets have been domesticated and kept as pets for over 2000 years; in fact, the first recorded domesticated Ferret belonged to none other than Julius Caesar, the Roman Emperor. They were originally domesticated as working animals, and used to hunt rabbits and the like, and are still employed in this way today, as well as for pest control. Being a therapy animal is new territory for Ferrets, and helps improve the poor reputation that they sometimes have.

Unleashing the healing power of animals

Ferrets are great fun to be around, too! They are playful animals, who enjoy interacting with people, even wagging their tails and 'dooking' (a particular noise that all Ferrets make, which sounds extremely cute!) when they get excited. (It's a massive privilege if your Ferret wags their tail at you.) I could spend hours playing with my Ferret – he really brightens my day!

Ferrets are also intelligent ... and crafty, which makes for a rascally combination, as they will steal things and hide them, when no-one's looking, and are especially fond of rubber! The collective term for Ferrets is a 'business' and, given how crafty they are, I can easily imagine them organised as a 'business' in the true sense of the word, making a big profit!

Johnnie had all of his species' idiosyncrasies! He was fun, playful, cheeky, sneaky, and sleepy (sounds like we are renaming the Seven Dwarfs!); he had the ferrety odour, too, and if needed, the desire to kill. All domestic animals, whether or not we like it, retain their instinctive fight or flight reflex, and natural desire to survive. Johnnie was not vicious – far from it – but I have learned to always be aware of an animal's body language, and what it is saying. If threatened, an animal will automatically revert to survival mode, and this is something we should remember.

Johnnie was a good Ferret with an astounding temperament. We don't know the full story of his life before we met him, because, like all of the animals featured in this book, he was a rescue, but he came to us via a friend, Will, who owns a zoo. Will's zoo is in the middle of the countryside, in Telford, and has a long driveway that leads to the car park. One morning, at the end of this long driveway, he found a cardboard box, inside which was a Ferret, who was Johnnie. The Ferret was friendly, had obviously spent much time around people, and seemed well fed and cared for. What was not so obvious was why he had been dumped on the doorstep of a zoo ...

Johnnie was introduced to the zoo's resident Ferret population, although it transpired that he had not been socialised with other Ferrets, and knew only humans! Not being one to give up easily – and noticing that this Ferret was quite a pleasant little chap – my friend persisted in trying to integrate Johnnie into his zoo business, and did so for months, but to no avail: Johnnie and the other Ferrets simply did not get on. This was when we got the phone call.

I had known Will and his wife, Becky, for a while, and we had visited each other's establishments numerous times, allowing us to see how each worked, and develop both a business and social relationship. When it was obvious that Johnnie was not going to adapt to life with others of his kind, Will immediately thought of us, as a Ferret was an animal that we did not have ... which made us the ideal home for a Ferret who did not like to be around other Ferrets. Will explained Johnnie's story to me, much as I have explained it here, and asked if we would like to add him to our critters for educational experience and therapy work, because he thought that Johnnie would be perfect for it. Of course, I said 'Yes' without hesitation.

After putting down the phone, I set about creating space for Johnnie in our house, and under the stairs was the ideal location. I was extremely lucky to have a very understanding landlord, who allowed me to keep animals, and the understairs cupboard was ideal for Johnnie: big enough to allow him to run around; high enough to allow him to climb: he had pipes and platforms and a hammock swinging high. I also provided him with a ball-pit which he loved to just lie in, once he had dived in to check it for treats!

Johnnie arrived a few days later, and was an instant hit. Will and Becky introduced him to us, and watched as we got to know each other; Johnnie had us all in hysterics: he was such a fun and characterful animal, with a heart of gold. Jean (my ex-wife) and three stepchildren all adored him, as he was playful and gentle, and not at all how Ferrets usually behave (there was no biting). He had obviously been loved at some stage, and been a massive part of somebody's family, because he loved being a part of ours from the moment he arrived. It was almost as though he felt he was back where he belonged.

After my friends left, Johnnie set off to explore the house, checking out every nook and cranny he could find, and memorising the best places that he would return to and use for rest and relaxation! He also checked out the other critters he met on his way, especially the cats and dogs. He got the usual reaction from the cats – nose-in-the-air disdain as they jumped past him, pretending he wasn't there. Johnnie would turn to go after them, but then run along sideways in the direction he was already going, 'dooking' away to himself. The dogs, on the other hand, were a little less sure of themselves around him, appearing a little nervous of their new companion, even though Johnnie wasn't particularly interested in them.

Johnnie found two places that he especially seemed to enjoy hiding in – the cats' baskets in our laundry room and my motorcycle helmet! I didn't have a motorcycle at the time, and I only remembered that Johnnie used to sleep in the helmet when I bought a motorcycle recently and needed the helmet – Johnnie's fur and scent were still there, flooding me with favourite memories of him, like the time I opened the wardrobe door to find him curled up tightly in the helmet, fast asleep and gently snoring!

Johnnie was a great asset in therapy work because he always did one very important thing – he made people smile – a lot! That is not only important when entertaining, but also when educating. Smiling helps children to retain information, because if learning is fun, they will learn more readily. In therapy, smiles and laughter are beneficial, too, because, as Charles Darwin stated in 1872: "The free expression by outward signs of emotion intensifies it." We automatically feel happier when we smile (which some psychologists call the 'facial feedback hypothesis'), and my

Unleashing the healing power of animals

JOHNNIE FEELGOOD
Speaking at a conference in 2016, I was addressing a room full of psychologists, specialists, and other mental health professionals about the value of the work I do. I began by asking all of those who had pets to stand up.

I then made this simple statement: "If your pet does not leave you feeling positive, please sit down." Everyone, remained standing, and I realised I had a room full of people who were going to totally understand the benefits of my work.

view and experience is that animals make people feel happier simply by their presence (assuming, of course, that the person in question likes animals).

Johnnie the smile-maker was relatively old (four or five) when he arrived with us. The lifespan of a Ferret is only seven or eight years, and he did give me a few scares, in terms of his health. On one occasion, when the weather was particularly hot, despite having frozen bottles of water in his enclosure and a house that was cool, he became quite lame, so I rushed him to the vet to be told he was suffering from heat exhaustion. After an injection, and electrolyte solution to rehydrate him, thankfully, he was back to the old Johnnie I knew and loved. This was a lesson in how important it is to ensure our furry friends remain cool in warmer months: even with all of the cooling aids provided, Johnnie still succumbed to the heat.

The biggest scare I had was when Johnnie stopped eating. As already mentioned, he liked to explore the house, and during the hours that people were about, Johnnie had free reign there. Mostly he could be found fast asleep in my motorcycle helmet, or in a cat bed in the laundry, but, on this particular day, he stayed within his enclosure under the stairs. It was obvious he was under the weather as he simply wasn't his usual self. He hadn't eaten his breakfast, and was not keen to come out and play as he usually was. Once again, I took him straight to the vet who had a feel around, administered an injection, and gave me some electrolyte solution and a syringe. He instructed me to give Johnnie a syringe-full of the solution every couple of hours, keep a close eye on him, and see if he had improved the next day.

I spent the afternoon, evening, and all night nursing Johnnie as he just laid on my lap. When it was time for his syringe he accepted it bravely and then went back to sleep. An obvious thing I noticed was that nothing was coming out of Johnnie: he was neither urinating or defecating. First thing the next morning we were straight back to the vet, who kept Johnnie in this time to do x-rays and various tests to ascertain what the problem was. The results showed that Johnnie had eaten an entire pencil eraser, which had become stuck in his stomach at the exit to his intestines: an emergency operation was needed to remove it. The vet had done a great job of identifying the problem, and the operation went well, especially given that Johnnie was no longer a youngster at around seven years of age. Suffice to say, access to the children's rooms was restricted for Johnnie after that, and all doors were kept closed when he was out and about!

All the time he had been with us Johnnie had been attending therapy sessions at the psychiatric hospitals I visited (where he earned the nickname 'Febreeze' because of his musky odour), and residential care homes. He was very popular at the hospitals because of his playful and mischievous nature, and the fact that he made everyone smile and giggle. He was so trustworthy it was possible to let him play out in the hospital garden when the weather permitted, giving him much freedom during sessions, and where patients could not only play with him, but also walk him. Walking an animal teaches responsibility and care towards other living things, as well as provide exercise for patients who otherwise might not do so.

In residential care homes Johnnie was popular simply because he was a Ferret. Ferret ownership is currently on the rise in the UK, especially amongst young, upper class women, but it was also extremely popular from the 1950s to the 1970s. Like tortoises, Ferrets were often a family pet, as well as working animals on farms, helping to provide dinner – a rabbit or two – for the family. A 'sport' popular at that same time was 'Ferret-legging,' in which competitors' trousers were tied at the ankle and a live Ferret introduced into the top of the trousers. The winner was the last competitor to release the Ferret from their trousers, and the world record stands at five hours and 30 minutes.

I have held a Ferret for five minutes or more on several occasions, and I can tell you they are wriggly at best, so really cannot imagine having a Ferret in my trousers for five or more hours. But I have met men in residential care homes who have competed, and who remember these times, and they derive great pleasure from recounting their stories and reliving the memories. And both male and female residents recount stories of 'ferreting' (hunting) with their fathers in the thirties and forties to find food for the Lord of the Manor, his family and staff. At one time it was only the wealthy who were allowed to keep Ferrets for hunting purposes, so some were illegally kept by poachers, and I have met men and women whose fathers were poachers. It's right that neither of these activities continues today, for the sake of the Ferrets, but Johnnie revived fond memories, smiles and joyful tears for those in care homes we visited.

Sadly, all good things must come to an end, and Johnnie inevitably succumbed to old age at around seven-and-a-half years of age. Always, the worst part of living with and caring for animals is having to say goodbye. Working with my animals so closely every day means that we laugh together and love together, forming a special bond in each case and becoming very close. And some curl up in a special place in my heart, and will remain there for the rest of my life. Johnnie was one of these, and I was heartbroken when he died. As with Mooch, I cried for days, but eventually found solace in the joy he gave to the countless people he met over the years; he will always be remembered with a smile.

After he had passed on, with Will and Becky we buried Johnnie's ashes in the zoo's Garden of Remembrance, reserved for the most special of the zoo's animals. This was a fine and fitting honour for Johnnie, which I am sure he would have been very proud of.

11
And then there are 'The Others'

Many animals work with me in the therapy sessions and educational work I do, most of whom are rescues. A small number are not, however, but if I was to write a chapter on each of them, this book would have more pages than *War and Peace*, so I've combined them in this, the last chapter about my animals.

'The Others' is a good way to categorise these as there are 'other' Snakes, 'other' Lizards, 'other' Rabbits; a new Ferret, and 'other' Hedgehogs. But there are also Frogs and insects and Skunks – yes, Skunks! – and all of these are therapy animals, too.

Let me introduce you to a couple of the more unusual ones, and explain how they help people.

The beneficial effects of furry animals in therapy are well documented, and, hopefully by now, you will also appreciate how other, not so obviously appealing, animals such as snakes and lizards can help, too. So what about insects? That's right, insects: creepy crawly creatures who frequently inspire fear, loathing, and disgust ... and that itchy feeling we get when we think something is dirty!

"Insects aren't animals!" I hear you cry ... but I would beg to differ.

The dictionary definition of an animal is –
'a living organism which feeds on organic matter, typically having specialised sense organs and a nervous system, and able to respond rapidly to stimuli.'

– and so, by its very definition, an insect *is* an animal: not only do they eat organic matter, they also respond to stimuli and feel pain.

Insects carry a stigma all their own – as do mental health issues – and patients and individuals with issues such as these relate to insects because of this, leaping to the animals' defence if anybody says something negative about them. Insects are not obviously appealing in the looks department, but study them closely for a while, and you may well see things you've not noticed before – their eyes are beautiful; their component parts are fascinating; their colours are amazing. There is even more to see and appreciate when you open your minds and your heart to them. Nature is magical in all her beauty, and never more evident than when we look at how insects work.

Tarantulas, Stick Insects and Millipedes are some of the insects in my team. The Tarantulas are mainly for clients with phobias, but are also what I term a 'technical' animal; of particular fascination to those with high level autism, because of the many parts that comprise the animal, not to mention what goes on inside them. Stick Insects are, again, a technically-fascinating animal, and because they are harmless, they are easier to study as it's possible to get much closer to them – 'user-friendly' indeed!

I frequently include Millipedes in my sessions, because they are also a sensory animal, although I cannot take the credit for realising the significance of this in therapy work, as this came from my lovely friend, Carrie Alcock. Carrie owns and runs a company called Rent a Beast, which focuses on educating children about the wonders of 'mini beasts.' We were in attendance at the National Pet Show at Stoneleigh, helping on Dr Daniel Allen's 'Pet Nation' stand, and chatting about my work, and how I used Stick Insects and Tarantulas. Carrie asked if I had ever thought about using Millipedes as a sensory therapy animal, handing me an outsize example of some 6-8 inches in length. I was a little cautious about handling the animal at first, but soon became fascinated.

Carrie told me all about them and, just like the little fellow with hundreds of legs, I was hooked! The Millipede's legs felt incredible on my skin, as they moved just like a Mexican wave rippling down the creature's length. The bugs crawling on the Millipede in symbiotic union (the Millipede provides them with a home; they clean the Millipede) simply added to the fascination. I use Millipedes mainly with children, although they are also very popular with my psychiatric hospital patients. How a Millipede feels on the skin can be likened to how Velcro works. This has a soft surface and a hard surface which stick together, and, when pulled apart, a resistance is felt. The legs of a Millipede represent the hard surface and our skin represents the soft surface: when gently lifting a Millipede from skin, the same sort of resistance is experienced.

A light ticklish, prickly feeling is felt when a Millipede walks on skin, similar to pins and needles. To sensitive skin, the movement of a Millipede can be quite intense, and to an autistic person with hypersensitive skin, it can be incredibly painful and almost impossible to bear, causing much distress. Holding hands, hugging a loved one, for example, and even the lightest touch, becomes impossible ... but Millipedes can help alleviate this hypersensitivity.

Short exposure in repeated bursts to contact with a Millipede – placed on the skin for just a second and then removed until the person has recovered from the contact – can gradually acclimatise them to touch. The patient alone decides when and for how long this happens – it's very similar to exposure therapy for phobias. At each session the time that the Millipede is on the patient's skin is increased a little, in accordance with what he or she feels comfortable with, and recovery becomes shorter.

Eventually, the patient is happy for the insect to crawl on their skin for a good amount of time, at which stage, immediately following the session with the Millipede, it is possible for a parent to stroke their skin, hold their hand, and even hug them. In many cases, this will be the first ever physical interaction between parent and child in a long time, and possibly even ever! As I expect you can imagine, this is an emotional experience for everybody concerned.

The more treatment is carried out, the more desensitized the skin will become. Not bad for a humble insect, eh? Luckily, children do not tend to feel the fears and prejudices that adults often do.

From an insect, we move to a furry animal, and probably one of the most notorious creatures ever to have walked the planet – the Skunk. The animal's Latin name is mephitis mephitis (mephitis meaning 'noxious' or 'foul smelling'); a smell which is that bad they had to name him twice! Native Indians called the animal 'shee-gawk' which is the basis for the word Chicago, meaning 'Skunk-land.'

It's generally thought that Skunks smell bad, and particularly so if they feel threatened, giving them an undeserved reputation for being obnoxious creatures. But Flower, the Skunk in the Disney film Bambi, is a far more accurate representation of what a Skunk is really like: sweet, beautiful, unassuming creatures, with no more intention of creating a stink than have you or I.

The smell in question comes from a liquid that the animal squirts from two glands situated just beneath the anus ... but only if the animal fears for their life, and even then only after giving several warnings. So, to debunk one myth, it is this liquid that smells and not the Skunk, who is actually one of the cleanest animals I've ever encountered. Many people (and especially children) are under the impression that the smell is created because the Skunk breaks wind, which is absolutely *not* the case. My maxim is 'If you are nice to the Skunk, then the Skunk will be nice to you!' and, although I appreciate that the behaviour of wild Skunks and domestic Skunks differs hugely, one of my ambitions is to go to America with a film crew and spend time with wild Skunks, to prove this.

As far as I am aware, I am the first animal assisted therapy practitioner in the UK – if not the world – to use a Skunk in a true therapy situation. Neither of my Skunks – Stoosh and Skittles – has had their scent glands removed (it is illegal to do so in England, in any case), and so are 'fully loaded,' and could spray anybody, at any time. Stoosh is my main therapy Skunk, as she is the most laidback of the two. I do occasionally work with Skittles, but more on a one-to-one basis as this is what she is most comfortable with.

The stigma associated with a Skunk can be both a disadvantage and advantage. One of the reasons people with mental health issues respond to them is because they empathise with others judging them on how they perceive them. A Skunk carries a stigma, as does mental illness, and so, immediately, there is the beginning of a bond. Unlike insects, however, Skunks are furry, with pretty faces, and they make us smile. Because of their obvious cuteness, the animal's stigma is usually forgotten.

Pretty soon, those receiving therapy begin to realise what awesome animals Skunks really are, and they become extremely defensive of Stoosh, for example, toward anyone who exhibits any form of prejudice.

Being very sweet animals – affectionate, laidback and peaceful most of the time – much like Cats, Skunks will happily sleep on a lap for as long as you want, pretty much, and seem to consider it a great honour (unlike cats!). This is what Stoosh will do, anyhow.

In fact, I stopped using Cats as therapy animals because I found they could have a detrimental effect on peoples' self-esteem, because everything has to be done on their terms. Cats do not especially like change – or strangers – so placing them in a situation they find uncomfortable is not good for either cat or patient.

For example, I might lift a Cat from their carrier and place him or her on the lap of a patient, whereupon the Cat jumps off the lap and climbs back into the carrier, prompting the inevitable reaction "Oh, she doesn't like me!" with accompanying sad expression and negative body language. Allowing a Cat to simply wander the room is not terribly successful either, as, more often than not, the animal will usually ignore an outstretched hand and dive back into the carrier, prompting a similarly crestfallen reaction from the patient, who is already struggling with self-esteem issues.

But, Stoosh, on the other hand, is the complete opposite, eliciting the delighted response: "She loves me, doesn't she? She's gone straight to sleep on me." Skunks are also very warm and fluffy, just perfect for releasing those feel good hormones in the brain, reducing heart rate and blood pressure, and, as they are so warm, providing the added benefit of spreading warmth through a patient's legs and stomach, just like a hot water bottle! I had one patient – a paranoid schizophrenic – who, when he spent time with Stoosh, said that the voices in his head stopped. For the hour's duration of each session, and a short while after, his head was blessedly free of its usual cacophony, giving him the opportunity to talk to others, such as his psychologist, calmly and with clarity.

I am very lucky with Stoosh, inasmuch as she is, and always has been, extremely calm, and at her happiest when with people. My other Skunk, Skittles, not so much, and my theory to explain this is that Stoosh was born and raised in a house with other animals and people close by all of the time, whereas Skittles was born and raised in an outdoor enclosure, without the same close and constant exposure to people and other animals, giving her more of a 'wild' nature. The best therapy Skunks will therefore be those who have been domesticated from a very young age, having close contact with people.

We have also had a couple of other really special cases using Skunks within a therapeutic environment. Both were patients at psychiatric hospitals: we'll call them 'Patient A' and 'Patient B.'

Patient A used to come to group sessions when I first began doing these. He would walk into the session, look at the animals with interest, and then walk out shaking his head. He never remained in a session. About a year later, the first time I introduced Stoosh in a therapy session, this patient walked in and did his usual scan of the animals, but this time something caught his eye. Patient A stopped at Stoosh's carrier, his face beamed, and he sat on the sofa patting his lap excitedly (instead of speaking he would simply gesture). We asked what it was he wanted, and he pointed to the carrier holding Stoosh, then patted his lap.

I duly placed Stoosh on his lap, and explained to him how she liked to be stroked: long, firm strokes. Stoosh happily settled on his lap and went to sleep, as the patient calmly stroked her for around an hour, and then indicated that he was ready to leave. I took Stoosh from his lap, thanked him, gave her a kiss, and placed her back in her carrier. Around 45 minutes later, Patient A approached me wearing a big smile, and holding a piece of paper which he passed to me. The paper had a drawing on it, of him sitting on the sofa with a Skunk on his lap, which he wanted me to have (unfortunately, this was not permitted).

It was Stoosh's very first therapy session, and one of my most memorable. Patient A continued to come to every therapy session and enjoy time with Stoosh, eventually actually talking to me about her and other things. A very successful debut for what is now an established therapy animal.

Patient B (who was originally permanently confined to a wheelchair) is a more recent success story. Suffering with depression, and not able to communicate well due to a brain injury, this person likes all animals, and attends every session.

Within just a few sessions, it was obvious Stoosh was a clear favourite amongst the animals, and he would sit with her resting along his thigh, stroking her and talking to her. Because of his difficulty with communication, he sometimes has to repeat what he says many, many times when talking with another person, but this wasn't necessary at all with Stoosh. Patient B has become truly attached to Stoosh, and feels a certain degree of ownership towards her (not uncommon); he even has a picture of her on his wall. If Stoosh does not appear at a session for any reason, it really does upset him. The beauty of this relationship is that clarity of speech does not matter to Stoosh, but, by talking to her, Patient B is practicing talking, developing speech patterns and, hopefully, improving his oral communication.

In addition to this, Patient B has learnt, from discussions we have had, that it is possible to walk a Skunk on a leash, which has inspired him to do something truly remarkable: get out of his wheelchair and learn to walk again! He is currently going to the hospital gym and cycling for around ten minutes a day to build strength in his legs. And exercise, as we know, also releases endorphins that will help combat his depression, and give him motivation to move forward.

His ultimate goal – his dream – is to walk Stoosh around the hospital grounds, and this happy event really cannot come soon enough for him. He has the drive and determination to achieve this, thanks to his bond with Stoosh: extraordinary Skunk, therapy animal, and his inspiration. This is a beautiful example of the benefits of unleashing the healing power of animals.

Another case in which Stoosh made a significant difference also involved a brain-injured patient. When I got to this patient one day, she was in the grip of a full body tremor, and showing signs of distress. I placed Stoosh on her lap and then arranged her hands so that one rested on Stoosh's back, so that she could feel her fur, placing the other on the arm of the special chair she was sitting in. Within minutes, the distressing tremors had subsided to virtually nothing, allowing the patient to close her eyes and drift off to sleep, along with Stoosh who had already dozed off! A combination of Stoosh's reassuring weight, the comfort of her body warmth and relaxed breathing had soothed the troubled patient sufficiently to allow sleep to come.

And there are a great many other animals, exotic and otherwise, who would make fabulous therapy animals. Horses are proven to have therapeutic value, for example, and I'm also sure that Goats, Sheep and Pigs do, too. I have considered trying other exotic creatures – such as Coatimundi, Meerkats, and Raccoons – although, after careful research and investigation, have decided against these, mainly because of how their temperament might develop upon maturity. If I had the funds I would love to try working with an Armadillo. I have done the groundwork, and this species seems suitable for therapy work.

The satisfaction I derive from seeing people positively interacting with my animals, and reaping the benefits of doing so, is second to none. I cannot imagine anything better than helping somebody who is in a bad place find peace and contentment, even if only for an hour.

I am really proud of my animals. Watching them with people, and seeing how amazingly tolerant and understanding they are, and the reactions of those they help, makes me fall in love with them all over again.

Animals are both amazing and wonderful. They expect nothing, yet unconditionally give their all, and this is their healing power. In this, I am merely a facilitator, whose job it is to unleash that power: the healing power of animals.

And then there are 'The Others'

I hope you've enjoyed reading my book,
We've talked about rescues, and had a good look,
At all of the animals with therapy skills,
Be these critters with fur, scales, hard shells or quills.

We've looked at these animals, and many more
Who weren't rescues; they just arrived at our door!
We have a relationship, strong, tried and true
So we can relay our therapy to you.

There are many animals in this world where we live
Who, without even trying, are ready to give.
By being with nature, we can readily see
The world has its own form of assistance therapy.

If animals can live in peace and just be,
Then why, on this beautiful Earth, can't we ...?

Epilogue

A dog called Beanz came to stay,
And I never want him to go away.
He's warm and furry, and fiercely loyal
With an intense affection that makes me feel royal.

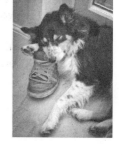

A playful boy who can run amok
Rounding up his imaginary flock,
Running round in circles grand
Covering every inch of land.

The only sounds he ever makes
Are in his dreams, but when he wakes,
He's the quietest dog, who doesn't say 'ruff'
I guess it's down to all his 'stuff.'

What he's been through, I will never know,
But I'll take him with me wherever I go.
No more bad times will he ever see
I'll keep him close: he's a part of me.

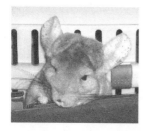

Soft and silky, with fur so fine
Came hopping over to live at mine.
His face so cute, with big brown eyes
It was love at first sight, I can't deny.

A Chinchilla boy, what can I say?
When he came to me, he came to stay,
He wasn't happy with human touch
But I wanted to sit and stroke him so much.

Epilogue

Like everything, with time it came
Patience and love would see him tame.
His popularity grew and grew
And this Sebastian quickly knew.

He shakes his whiskers and hops about
Then, with his paw, he wipes his snout.
He sits and watches, and doesn't stir
Whilst his biggest fans gently caress his fur.

A special boy, with personality to match,
He's quick on his feet and hard to catch,
But every day we chat for a while
And every day he makes me smile.

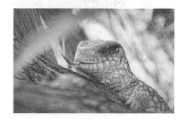

You came to us from far away;
We brought you home here to stay.
So beautiful, I stood in awe,
As I watched you roam and explore.

Who could have known
How we would grow?
Something special between us two
I loved the time I spent with you.

Side by side we'd show them how,
We'd make them laugh and make them 'WOW!'
You did your bit and I did mine,
If only we'd had a little more time.

Over time we built up trust,
A love, a union, a lifetime must,
I'd hug you and you'd hug me,
A bond that everyone could see.

Today you left, it was your time,
To leave your family behind.
We held your hand, and cried and cried,
We felt a love so deep inside.

One last hug I thought I'd share
To show for you my love and care,
To help you on your journey far,
To help you shine – the brightest star.

Unleashing the healing power of animals

Good luck, my Mooch, in lives to come,
To give love and warmth just like the sun.
Memories remain to make me smile,
Remember me, too, once in a while.

Bon voyage, Mooch – we love you x

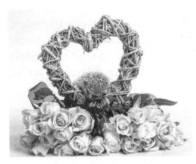

The time you had after you were born,
Was not a time that was the norm.
Passed from pillar to similar post,
Eventually, you got a home to boast.

Two lovely people to treat you well
And save you from a domestic hell.
They gave you toys and lots of space,
They gave you love; your life was ace!

Despite being spoiled, you could not see,
So their grumpy hog was christened Wasabi.
Your sharp, stiff spines just would not yield
Like a wild hedgehog, in a wild green field.

They tried and tried, but to no avail
So, when the time was right, you moved in with Dale.
He continued their work and brought you round,
Until you were happy to be out, with no protest sound.

You worked in therapy for a year or two,
And those you met fell in love with you.
Sometimes you'd play and make people shout 'Yikes!'
As they felt the sharp ends of your prickly spikes!

A white snake, found in a field,
Nothing there you could use as a shield.
A fox, a badger, a predatory bird,
All of which could pick you off, unheard.

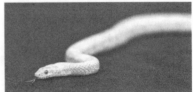

Before anything could happen to you,
You were spotted there, and picked up, too.
You were the most beautiful snake in the grass,
But when gathered up, you showed your sass.

You were in a box, when we first met.
I hadn't decided whether to keep you, yet,
But after some time, it became quite clear
That you and I had a future to share.

Frostie, the Snow Corn, a Christmas snake
Was the debut you were meant to make,
And there and then you became a star,
Just a few years later, you've come so far.

How many you've helped ... I've lost count,
But I know for sure it's a large amount.
So many people, both young and old
Continues to increase, by ten-fold.

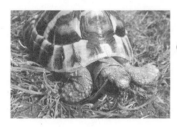

You arrived with us when you were small,
But soon captured the hearts of one and all.
George, you're a character who belies his size,
And wisdom and mischief shine in your eyes.

Around the house, you make your way
Exercising nearly every day.
When the door is open wide,
You take eager steps to venture outside.

One afternoon I remember well,
(Although I swore I would never tell),
Creeping up slowly to a black, wet nose
You bit with force, high on your toes.

Poor old Beanz, jumped outta his skin,
Fast asleep when you dived in!
He had no idea what was going on,
As you sauntered by ... and wandered on.

The effect you have on those you meet,
Is nothing short of a miraculous feat,
You induce calmness, love and smiles
And bring back memories that were gone awhile.

To you, dear George, we raise a glass
To the many miracles you will amass,
Smiles galore and memories, too,
We look forward to sharing them all with you!

Unleashing the healing power of animals

Tinkerbell, a rabbit lop
Whose long ears don't stand up, but flop.
A fluffy bun, with the softest fur,
Whose start in life was bad for her.

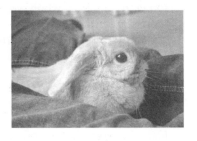

Unkindly mated, from an early age,
Never leaving her breeding cage;
Having litters, one, two, three,
A sad, sad start to her family tree.

We came along, took her away,
To give her love and help her play;
To care for her as best we could,
As anyone with feelings would.

As time went by, and Tink did grow,
A beautiful soul this girl did show,
A soul so deep and so sublime
For therapy, it was now time.

And so she joined, a huge success,
A big surprise, I must confess;
To see her reach and nudge a chin
Sensing something deep within.

She makes the day for young and old,
Turning warm what once was cold.
"Thank you, Tinks," they always say,
"Oh, Tinkerbell, come back and play!"

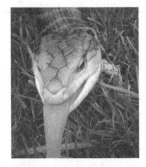

A Scale of Two Cities, the title suggests
Through travel and need, your tale manifests;
A need for care that is proper and true,
A need for a carer, looking out just for you.

Through time spent together, sorting you out;
Giving you everything, you wanted for nowt;
We developed a bond that brought us real close,
So much so you were soon kissing my nose!

A beautiful lady with tongue of a hue
A rich, penetrating, wonderful blue.

Epilogue

You fascinate people with just how you are,
A cold-blooded, reptilian, critterish star!

People who sit with you instantly calm,
Be you on their lap or resting on an arm.
Sitting so still, you enjoy all of their strokes,
Everyone smiles; some laugh, and some joke!

The life you now lead is better than twas,
You get all that you want and are happy because
You've no need to worry, wherever you go,
You will meet only friend, and never a foe.

Johnnie was a ferret, abandoned in a box
At the end of a road, strewn about with rocks.
When the box was opened, he jumped right on out,
With an expression that said "What's this all about?"

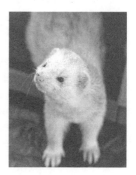

The people who found him, they lived in a zoo
And straight away they knew just what to do
"We'll put him with our lot, it'll be the 'business,'"
they said
And to the ferret enclosure they quickly sped.

But all of the effort and best will in the world,
Could not make Johnnie like a boy ferret, or girl.
They tried for a while, then came up with a plan,
They'd deliver him to the Critterish Allsorts Man!

The day Johnnie arrived he was a bundle of joy,
A happy-go-lucky, ferrety boy.
And so he remained; his character set,
Making such a difference to those he met.

He visited care homes, and hospitals, too,
He went in to schools; even back to the zoo!
He was Top of the Pops; a Number 1 hit!
With all of the patients he was the perfect fit.

Johnnie, you made me laugh, with a great big smile
That I wore with pride, you had such style.
You're one of my critters I will forever miss,
With your hop and your 'dook' – your ferret business!

Testimonials

- I have been involved in animal sessions with Dale many times, in two different school settings. Both schools are schools that work with students with 'Special Educational Needs,' predominantly Autism. Over the sessions I have witnessed the students light up at the prospect of handling the reptiles and other animals. Students engage with the animals, and have even developed communication skills that were unknown before the integration of the animals. Having witnessed the huge positive impact that this experience has on the students, I would say this experience could be one of the most positive, engaging, and worthwhile that students may ever have.
  – *Lewis Kirk, Assistant Head Teacher, Fox Hollies School, Birmingham*

- Knowing Dale and his work with animal assisted therapy for several years, I can honestly say the passion, knowledge and dedication he has for the welfare of his animals, and the people who are lucky enough to meet them, is nothing short of incredible. He has an infectious enthusiasm for life, a natural affinity for helping animals and humans in need, and is an absolute pleasure to work with.
  – *Sean McCormack BSc (Hons), MVB, MRCVS; Veterinary Surgeon*

- Dale's work through animal assisted therapy is an inspiration. During the years I have known him, Dale has repeatedly demonstrated how the healing that can take place when we connect with animals truly can transform lives. – *Lisa Tenzin-Dolma, Author, Principal, The International School for Canine Psychology and Behaviour; Founder of The Dog Welfare Alliance*

- Dale has been visiting the patients at our CAMHS Inpatient Unit every month for the past year. The patients always look forward to his visits, and spend a lot of time discussing and choosing which animals they would like him to bring. The day of the visit is always filled with excitement as they wait for Dale and his friends to arrive.

  The interaction between the animals and the patients is amazing and it has triggered responses in some, who have shown little or no interaction with staff or their peers up to that point. It also creates an air of calm across the ward which remains for some time after.

  The visits are always a pleasurable experience for both patients and staff, and we hope to continue these into the future.
  – *Jackie Hopkins, Activity Co-ordinator, CAMHS Inpatient Unit, Birmingham*

- Dale's work with my daughter and her phobia of dogs has been life-changing. She now loves dogs and is happy in their presence. In addition, she has become a more confident person, has greater self-esteem, and is much richer for the therapeutic experience that the sessions have provided her with.
  – *Gill Stanton, about the therapy her daughter received for cynophobia (Jan 2016 to August 2016)*

- Dale is an amazing animal guy! He shares his love for animals in such a sweet way that it is impossible for you not to love the animals as much as he does! He was able to teach my students to respect and love all animals. He created an atmosphere of genuine love of all animals. The life lessons were a bonus. We love Mr Dale!
  – *Bobbi Capwell, teacher (retired), Hall Elementary School and Greene Elementary School, League City, Houston, Texas, USA (visited via Skype and in person)*

- Working as a veterinary surgeon, I see on a daily basis how important pets are to human health and wellbeing. Dale and his colleagues (because that's what Stoosh, Skittles, Hoo, and all the other animals are) are the finest example I know of a team utterly dedicated to animal welfare and the human-animal bond.
  – *Dr Mark B Hedberg, The Expat Vet (www.expatvet.com)*

Patient comments
- "When I am with Stoosh [the Skunk], all of the noise in my head disappears."

- "It brings nature close to my heart and how I feel: like being content and peaceful in mind and body. It bought me a calmness."

Contact Dale Preece-Kelly –

Facebook: Critterish Allsorts
             Critter Assisted Therapy
             Dale Preece-Kelly (page)
Instagram: @critterman
             @dalepk_author
Twitter: @CritterishUK
             @DalePK_Author
             @therapyskunks

www.critterishallsorts.co.uk
www.critter-assisted-therapy.co.uk

Index

Abusive 56
Adults 11, 32, 43, 44, 75
Affection 9, 76, 80
Aggressive/aggression 5, 30, 56, 57
Animal assisted therapy 4, 6, 9-12, 17, 39, 42, 44, 56, 75, 86
Anxiety 12
Autism/autistic 4, 17, 74, 86

Behaviour 5, 11, 15, 20, 24, 25, 32, 61, 65, 75, 86
Benefits 4-6, 9, 18, 25, 27, 39, 44, 60, 61, 69, 70, 76, 78
Blood pressure 18, 76
Bond 5, 6, 9, 11, 21, 26, 28, 72, 76, 78, 81, 84, 87
Brain-injured 78
Business 6, 10, 12, 59, 60, 68, 85

Calm/calmness 4, 11, 18, 19, 24, 25, 31, 38, 44, 57, 61, 65, 66, 76, 77, 83, 85, 87
Care 5, 9-11, 14, 25, 36, 37, 41, 42, 61, 65, 71, 81, 84, 85
Care home 11, 16, 19, 23, 56, 71
Cat 9, 28, 31, 43, 54, 56, 69, 70, 76, 77
Child/children 8-11, 14, 15, 17, 21, 28, 30, 32, 35, 36, 39, 42-44, 55, 56, 59, 61, 69, 71, 74, 75
Chinchilla 4, 6, 21-26, 61, 80
CITES 53
Confidence/confident 9, 19, 20, 24, 32, 43, 44, 55, 58, 60, 67, 87
Connection 6, 9, 22, 25, 28, 57, 86

Dementia 16, 39, 56, 61
Depression 12, 43, 61, 62, 77, 78
Disabled 11, 42, 59
Dog 4, 7, 11, 13-20, 24, 29, 31, 32, 43, 54, 55, 69, 80, 86, 87

Education 6, 10, 36, 38, 41, 69, 73, 74, 86
Effects 24, 32, 43, 57, 61, 66, 73, 76, 83
Environment 4, 5, 25, 41, 55, 57, 61, 63-65, 77
Exotic 6, 9, 10, 19, 29, 65, 78

Ferret 6, 67-72, 73, 85

Happy 5, 8, 9, 14-16, 21, 23-26, 28-31, 38, 39, 42-44, 56, 58, 60, 61, 63, 65, 66, 75, 78, 80,
Healing 6, 11, 12, 78, 86
Health 4-6, 9-11, 26, 27, 29, 39, 61, 65, 70, 87
Heart rate 18, 76
Hedgehog 6, 35-39, 73, 82
Hormones 18, 32, 61, 76
Hospital 10, 16, 17, 19, 31, 32, 54, 71, 78, 85

Insects 4, 29, 73-76
Interacting/interaction 5, 11, 16, 18-20, 22, 23, 25, 44, 61, 62, 66-68, 75, 78, 87

License 53, 54
Lizard 6, 14, 28-33, 63-66, 73
Love 4, 5, 7-11, 15-18, 22-25, 31-33, 35, 37, 43, 53, 54, 57-61, 66, 69, 70, 72, 76, 78, 80-84, 87

Memory/memories 6, 8, 17, 24, 28, 39, 56, 69, 71, 82, 83
Mental health 4-6, 10-12, 26, 27, 39, 44, 59, 61, 66, 73, 76
Mental illness 11, 26, 76
Microchip 53-54

Oxytocin 18, 43

Patients 4-6, 11, 16-18, 21, 23, 24, 26, 27, 31, 32, 39, 42-44, 56, 57, 61, 62, 66, 71, 73-78, 86, 87
Pet 6, 7-9, 21, 22, 29, 30, 35-40, 53, 54, 56, 60, 67, 70, 71, 74, 87
Phobia 19, 20, 43, 74, 75, 87
Play 4, 16, 17, 19, 28, 30, 33, 36, 59, 67-71, 80, 82, 84
Practitioner 6, 11, 12, 75
Psychiatric hospital 10, 11, 16, 17, 19, 31, 32, 39, 42, 56, 61, 74, 77
Psychologist 6, 12, 26, 57, 61, 69, 70, 76
Psychosis 44, 66

Rabbit 6, 7-10, 30, 31, 58-62, 67, 71, 73, 84
Relationship 5, 6, 8, 11, 15, 20, 25, 28, 31-33, 36, 42, 44, 68, 77, 79

Relax/relaxed 4, 5, 20, 38, 43, 57, 61, 66, 69, 78
Reptile 4, 14, 19, 29, 32, 40, 41, 55, 66
Rescue/rescued 4, 11-15, 17, 18, 21, 25, 32, 35, 36, 40, 55, 58, 65, 68, 73, 79
Research 4, 7, 41, 65, 78
Residents 23-25, 56, 61, 68, 71
Responsibility 9, 71

Safety 5, 65
Schizophrenia/schizophrenic 4, 76
Schools 6, 10, 11, 19, 24, 55, 85-87
Self-esteem 4, 6, 8, 32, 43, 44, 66, 76, 87
Self-harm 26, 27
Serotonin 18, 43
Session 5, 16, 18, 26, 27, 32, 39, 42-44, 57, 60-62, 65, 66, 71, 73-77, 86, 87
Skunk 4, 6, 41, 67, 73, 75-78, 87
Smell 16, 30, 31, 34, 36-38, 55, 67, 75
Snake 6, 9, 14, 40-44, 63, 66, 73, 82, 83
Social/socially 6, 9, 38, 43, 58, 66, 68
Social skills 9
Stigma 42, 44, 73, 75, 76
Stroke/stroking 14, 16, 18, 19, 32, 33, 39, 43, 56, 61, 62, 65, 75, 77, 80, 85
Support 6, 11, 15, 35, 65

Temperament 5, 19, 20, 42, 44, 60, 65, 66, 68, 78
Therapeutic 4, 6, 17, 19, 25, 26, 77, 87
Therapy 4-6, 9, 11, 16-18, 20, 21-23, 31, 32, 38, 39, 42-44, 56, 57, 59-62, 65-67, 69, 71, 73-79, 82, 84, 86, 87
Tortoise 6, 53-57, 62, 71
Training 11, 14, 15, 21
Treatment, treated 8, 12, 21, 26, 35, 36, 56, 59, 64, 75
Trust, trusting 5, 11, 17, 22-25, 28, 31, 38, 54, 71, 81

Vet 5, 8, 33, 54, 59, 65, 70, 71, 86, 87